Essentials of Lung Cancer

With Orthodox and Alternative Treatment

Preface

I have written this book so that the patients suffering from Lung cancer can understand the disease in detail and choose a suitable treatment for them. This book provides detailed information about the clinical symptoms, complications, diagnosis, staging and treatments. In the last 15 years there has been considerable research and progress in the field of clinical studies, etiology, pathology, diagnosis and treatment of Lung cancer. Today we have new medicines, which work in a better way.

In this book, I have written in detail about Orthodox and Alternative Treatment (Budwig Protocol, which is the best alternative treatment and gives authentic success). Patient can carefully select the right treatment for him. This book has up to date information.

Dr. O.P.Verma

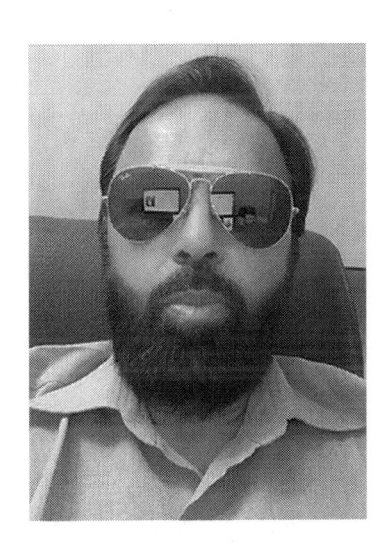

Written by
Dr. O.P. Verma
M.B.B.S., M.R.S.H. (London)
Budwig Wellness
7-B-43, Mahaveer Nagar III, Kota (Raj.)
+919460816360

I dedicate this book to my bosom friend Anil Paul. He is a very loving and sweet buddy. He is recently diagnosed Adenocarcinoma of lung. I know he will review all possible treatments in detail and will choose the best treatment for him. He is full of confidence and positivity. He will soon cure himself for sure. I pray to God for his happy, healthy and long life.

Dr. Om Verma

Copyright © 2019 by Dr. O.P.Verma
All rights reserved

Table of Content

Lung cancer 1
   Incidence 2
   Anatomy of the Lungs 2
   Blood Supply and Nervous Innervation of the Lungs 4
   Blood Supply 4
   Nerve supply to Lungs 5
   Pleura of the Lungs 5

Causes of Lung Cancer 7
   Oxygen deficiency is the prime cause 7
   Smoking 7
   Passive smoking 8
   Asbestos 8
   Radon gas 9
   Lung disease 9
   Prior history of lung cancer 10
   Air pollution 10
   Genetic 10

Types of Lung Cancer 11
   Small cell lung cancers (SCLC) 11
   Non-small cell lung cancers (NSCLC) 11
   Adenocarcinoma 12
   Squamous cell carcinomas 12
   Large cell carcinomas 13

Symptoms and signs 15
   No Symptoms 15
   Symptoms related to the cancer 15
   Symptoms related to metastasis 16
   Horner syndrome 16
   Superior vena cava syndrome 17
   Paraneoplastic syndromes 17

Diagnostic Workup 20
   History and clinical examination 20
   Chest X-ray 20
   CT scan (computerized tomography) 20
   MRI (Magnetic resonance imaging) 21
   Positron emission tomography (PET scanning) 21
   Bone scan 22
   Sputum cytology 23
   Bronchoscopy 23

Fine needle aspiration Cytology (FNAC) 25
Thoracentesis 25
Major surgical procedure 26
Laboratory Tests 26
Complete Blood Count (CBC) 27
Blood Chemistry Tests 27
Molecular Profiling (Genetic Testing) 28
Genetic Testing 29
What Are Gene Mutations? 29
Significance of Gene Mutations 30
Common Driver Mutations 31
Personalized Treatments 31
Tumor markers in lung cancer 33
Staging 37
Why Staging Is Important 37
TNM Staging 38
Treatment 42
Surgery 42
Radiotherapy 43
Chemotherapy 44
How Chemotherapy Works 45
How Chemotherapy Is Given 47
Medications 47
Why Can't Chemotherapy Cure Lung Cancer? 49
Side Effects of Chemotherapy 50
Photodynamic Treatment (PDT) 53
Radio Frequency Ablation (RFA) 54
Targeted Therapy 55
Lung Cancer Prognosis 61
Can Lung Cancer Be Prevented? 63
Alternative cancer treatments 66
Chemotherapy Doesn't Cure Cancer – It Causes It! 66
Laetrile (Vitamin B-17) Therapy 68
The Gerson Therapy 73
Simoncini's Baking Soda Cancer Treatment 76
Best Alternative Treatment - Budwig Protocol 77
Prime Cause of Cancer 80
Otto Warburg – Biography 80
Prime cause of Cancer 82
Dr. Johanna Budwig - Biography & Science 84
Budwig Protocol 91

Budwig Diet	92
Precautions	99
Prohibitions of Budwig Protocol	101
Few Desserts recipes by Dr. Budwig	103
ELDI oils	105
Coffee Enema	109
Epsom bath	112
Soda bicarb bath	113
Sun Therapy	113
Oil-Protein Diet while travelling	114
Making Quark	116
Making Cottage Cheese	116
Buckwheat	117
Energy Healing	119
How long should you take this protocol?	120
How do I recognize a good Flax seed oil?	121
Linomel	122
Questions and Answers	**123**
Budwig Diet & Protocol - In Brief	**125**
Lothar Hirneise	**128**
3E Program	130
Interview of Dr. Johanna Budwig	**133**
Sun, Photons and Electrons	**141**
Electrons	141
The sun's energy and man as an antenna	142
Fats Syndrome	144
Anti-Mensch	145
The electrons as resonance system	146
Daylight	148
Visualization - Path to wellness	**150**
Testimonials	**155**
Laetrile Testimonials	162
The Budwig Diet quotes	**164**
Disclaimer	**172**
My Books	**173**

Lung cancer

Lung cancer is an aggressive, widespread, and deadly disease, in which uncontrolled growth of lung tissues occurs. 90% to 95% of lung cancers originate from the epithelial cells of small and large respiratory tubules (bronchi and bronchioles). That is why it is also called bronchogenic carcinoma. The cancer caused by the lung's outer membrane (Plura) is called mesothelioma. Lung cancer spreads very quickly and it can spread to any part of the body. This is considered to be a very fatal disease. Its treatment is also very difficult.

Lung cancers are generally divided into two main categories: small cell lung cancer (SCLC) and non–small cell lung cancer (NSCLC). NSCLC accounts for approximately 85% of all lung cancers. Histologically, NSCLC is divided further into adenocarcinoma, squamous cell carcinoma (SCC), and large cell carcinoma.

Lung cancer was a rare entity in the early 1900s but has since become far more prevalent. The prevalence of lung cancer is second only to that of prostate cancer in men and breast cancer in women. By the end of the 1900s, lung cancer had become the leading cause of preventable death in the United States, and recently, it surpassed heart disease as the leading cause of smoking-related mortality.

Most lung carcinomas are diagnosed at an advanced stage, conferring a poor prognosis. The need to diagnose lung cancer at an early and potentially curable stage is thus important. In addition, most patients who develop lung cancer have been smokers and have smoking-related damage to the heart and lungs, making aggressive surgical or multimodality therapies less viable options.

Lung cancer is often insidious, producing no symptoms until the disease is well advanced. In approximately 7-10% of cases, lung cancers are diagnosed incidentally in asymptomatic patients, when a chest radiograph performed for other reasons reveals the disease. Numerous pulmonary signs may be associated with NSCLC. Systemic findings may include unexplained weight loss and low-grade fever.

Incidence

Lung cancer is the leading cause of cancer-related mortality in both men and women not only in the United States but also throughout the world. In 2016, the disease is expected to cause approximately 158,000 deaths in the United States—more than colorectal, breast, and prostate cancers combined. According to the National Cancer Institute, one in every 17 females and one in every 15 men develops lung cancer in their life time. The types of lung cancer in the United States, as well as in many other countries, have also changed in the past few decades: the frequency of adenocarcinoma has risen, and that of SCC has declined.

Lung cancer is often the disease of old age. Nearly 70% of patients are older than 65 years of age at diagnosis, only 3% of patients are younger than 45 years of age. Before 1930, this disease was very rare. But as the prevalence of cigarette smoking increased, the incidence of this disease has increased dramatically. These days, the incidence of this cancer has declined in many countries due to strict ban of smoking publicly, and health education. Nevertheless, lung cancer remains one of the leading cause of death in both men and women of the world.

Anatomy of the Lungs

A major organ of the respiratory system, each lung houses structures of both the conducting and respiratory zones. The main function of the lungs is to perform the exchange of oxygen and carbon dioxide with air from the atmosphere. To this end, the lungs exchange respiratory gases across a very large epithelial surface area—about 70 square meters—that is highly permeable to gases.

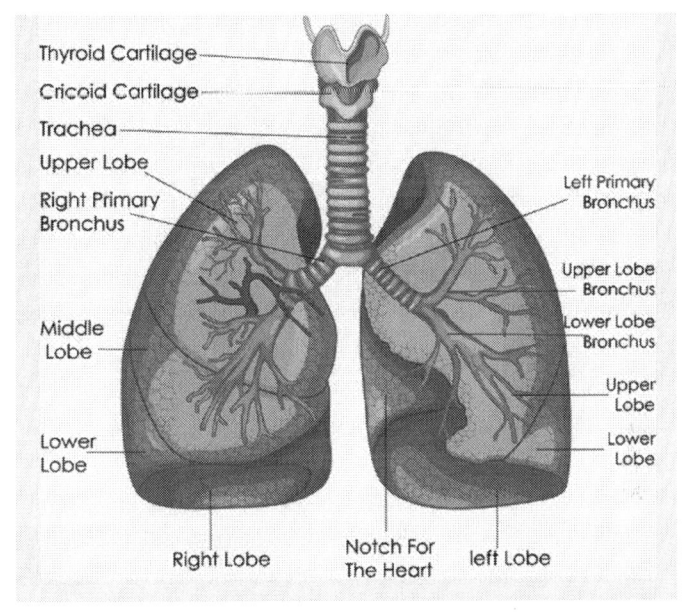

Figure labels: Thyroid Cartilage, Cricoid Cartilage, Trachea, Upper Lobe, Right Primary Bronchus, Middle Lobe, Lower Lobe, Left Primary Bronchus, Upper Lobe Bronchus, Lower Lobe Bronchus, Upper Lobe, Lower Lobe, Right Lobe, Notch For The Heart, left Lobe

    The lungs are pyramid-shaped, paired organs that are connected to the trachea by the right and left bronchi; on the inferior surface, the lungs are bordered by the diaphragm. The diaphragm is the flat, dome-shaped muscle located at the base of the lungs and thoracic cavity. The lungs are enclosed by the pleurae, which are attached to the mediastinum. The right lung is shorter and wider than the left lung, and the left lung occupies a smaller volume than the right. The cardiac notch is an indentation on the surface of the left lung, and it allows space for the heart. The apex of the lung is the superior region, whereas the base is the opposite region near the diaphragm. The costal surface of the lung borders the ribs. The mediastinal surface faces the midline.

    Each lung is composed of smaller units called lobes. Fissures separate these lobes from each other. The right lung consists of three lobes: the superior, middle, and inferior lobes. The left lung consists of two lobes: the superior and inferior lobes. A bronchopulmonary segment is a division of a lobe, and each lobe houses multiple bronchopulmonary segments. Each segment receives air from its own tertiary bronchus and is supplied with blood by its own artery. Some diseases of the lungs typically affect one or more bronchopulmonary segments, and in some cases, the diseased segments can be surgically removed with little influence on neighboring segments. A pulmonary lobule is a subdivision formed as the bronchi branch into bronchioles. Each lobule receives its own large bronchiole that has multiple branches. An interlobular septum is a wall, composed of connective tissue, which separates lobules from one another.

Blood Supply and Nervous Innervation of the Lungs

The blood supply of the lungs plays an important role in gas exchange and serves as a transport system for gases throughout the body. In addition, innervation by both the parasympathetic and sympathetic nervous systems provides an important level of control through dilation and constriction of the airway.

Blood Supply

The major function of the lungs is to perform gas exchange, which requires blood from the pulmonary circulation. This blood supply contains deoxygenated blood and travels to the lungs where erythrocytes, also known as red blood cells, pick up oxygen to be transported to tissues throughout the body. The pulmonary artery is an artery that arises from the pulmonary trunk and carries deoxygenated, arterial blood to the alveoli. The pulmonary artery branches multiple times as it follows the bronchi, and each branch becomes progressively smaller in diameter. One arteriole and an accompanying venule supply and drain one pulmonary lobule. As they near the alveoli, the pulmonary arteries become the pulmonary capillary network. The pulmonary capillary network consists of tiny vessels with very thin walls that lack smooth muscle fibers. The capillaries branch and follow the bronchioles and structure of the alveoli. It is at this point that the capillary wall meets the alveolar wall, creating the respiratory membrane. Once the blood is oxygenated, it drains from the alveoli by way of multiple pulmonary veins, which exit the lungs through the hilum.

Nerve supply to Lungs

Dilation and constriction of the airways are achieved through nervous control by the parasympathetic, and sympathetic nervous systems. The parasympathetic system causes bronchoconstriction, whereas the sympathetic nervous system stimulates bronchodilation. Reflexes such as coughing, and the ability of the lungs to regulate oxygen and carbon dioxide levels, also result from this autonomic nervous system control. Sensory nerve fibers arise from the vagus nerve, and from the second to fifth thoracic ganglia. The pulmonary plexus is a region on the lung root formed by the entrance of the nerves at the hilum. The nerves then follow the bronchi in the lungs and branch to innervate muscle fibers, glands, and blood vessels.

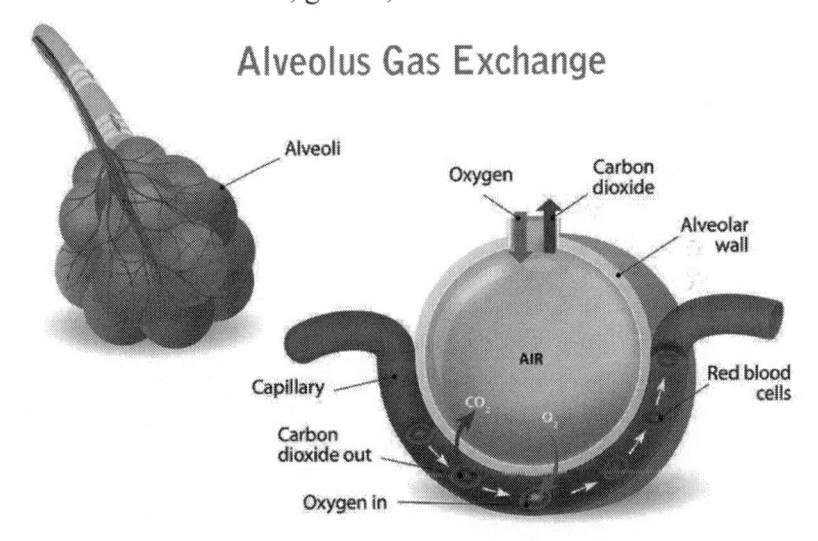

Pleura of the Lungs

Each lung is enclosed within a cavity that is surrounded by the pleura. The pleura (plural = pleurae) is a serous membrane that surrounds the lung. The right and left pleurae, which enclose the right and left lungs, respectively, are separated by the mediastinum. The pleurae consist of two layers. The visceral pleura is the layer that is superficial to the lungs, and extends into and lines the lung fissures. In contrast, the parietal pleura is the outer layer that connects to the thoracic wall, the mediastinum, and the diaphragm. The visceral and parietal pleurae connect to each other at the hilum. The pleural cavity is the space between the visceral and parietal layers.

The pleurae perform two major functions: They produce pleural fluid and create cavities that separate the major organs. Pleural fluid is secreted by mesothelial cells from both pleural layers and acts to lubricate their surfaces. This lubrication reduces friction between the two layers to prevent trauma during breathing, and creates surface tension that helps maintain the position of the lungs against the thoracic wall. This adhesive characteristic of the pleural fluid causes the lungs to enlarge when the thoracic wall expands during ventilation, allowing the lungs to fill with air. The pleurae also create a division between major organs that prevents interference due to the movement of the organs, while preventing the spread of infection.

Causes of Lung Cancer

Oxygen deficiency is the prime cause

Dr. Warburg summarized that all normal cells absolutely require oxygen, but cancer cells can live without oxygen - a rule without exception. Deprive a cell 35% of its oxygen for 48 hours and it would become cancerous. **Dr. Otto Warburg clearly mentioned that the root cause of cancer is lack of oxygen in the cells.**

He also discovered that cancer cells are anaerobic (do not breathe oxygen), get the energy by fermenting glucose and produce laevo-rotating lactic acid, and the body becomes acidic. Cancer cannot survive in the presence of high levels of oxygen, as found in an alkaline state.

He postulated that sulfur containing protein and some unknown fat is required to attract oxygen into the cell. **This fat plays a major role in the respiration and functioning of Warburg respiratory enzyme.**

Smoking

The incidence of lung cancer is strongly correlated with cigarette smoking, with about 90% of lung cancers arising as a result of tobacco use. The risk of lung cancer increases with the number of cigarettes smoked over time; doctors refer to this risk in terms of pack-years of smoking history (the number of packs of cigarettes smoked per day multiplied by the number of years smoked). For example, a person who has smoked two packs of cigarettes per day for 10 years has a 20 pack-year smoking history. While the risk of lung cancer is increased with even a 10 pack-year smoking history, those with 30 pack-year histories or more are considered to have the greatest risk for the development of lung cancer. Among those who smoke two or more packs of cigarettes per day, one in seven will die of lung cancer. But even though the risk is higher the more you smoke, there is no safe level of exposure to tobacco smoke.

Pipe and cigar smoking can also cause lung cancer, although the risk is not as high as with cigarettes. While someone who smokes one pack of cigarettes per day has a risk for the development of lung cancer that is 25 times higher than a nonsmoker. Pipe and cigar smokers have a risk of lung cancer that is about five times that of a nonsmoker.

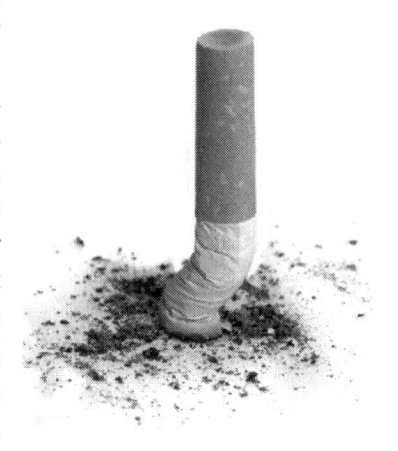

Tobacco smoke contains over 7,000 chemical compounds, many of which have been shown to be cancer-causing, or carcinogenic. The two primary carcinogens in tobacco smoke are chemicals known as nitrosamines and polycyclic aromatic hydrocarbons. The risk of developing lung cancer decreases each year following smoking cessation as normal cells grow and replace damaged cells in the lung. In former smokers, the risk of developing lung cancer begins to approach that of a nonsmoker about 15 years after cessation of smoking.

Passive smoking

The risk of this cancer is also 24% higher in those who live with smokers or spend long time with them than normal people. Of the patients, dying from lung cancer every year in the US, 3000 patients are from this category.

Asbestos

Asbestos fibers are silicate fibers that can persist for a lifetime in lung tissue following exposure to asbestos. The workplace is a common source of exposure to asbestos fibers, as asbestos was widely used in the past for both thermal and acoustic insulation materials. Today, asbestos use is limited or banned in many countries including the Unites States. Both lung cancer and mesothelioma (a type of cancer of the pleura or of the lining of the abdominal cavity called the peritoneum) are associated with exposure to asbestos. Cigarette smoking drastically increases the chance of developing an asbestos-related lung cancer in exposed workers. Asbestos workers who do not smoke have a fivefold greater risk of developing lung cancer than non-smokers, and those asbestos workers who smoke have a risk that is 50 to 90 times greater than non-smokers.

Radon gas

Radon gas is a natural, chemically inert gas that is a natural decay product of uranium. It decays to form products that emit a type of ionizing radiation. Radon gas is a known cause of lung cancer, with an estimated 12% of lung cancer deaths attributable to radon gas, or 15,000 to 22,000 lung cancer-related deaths occur annually in the U.S. As with asbestos exposure, concomitant smoking greatly increases the risk of lung cancer with radon exposure. Radon gas can travel up through soil and enter homes through gaps in the foundation, pipes, drains, or other openings. The U.S. Environmental Protection Agency estimates that one out of every 15 homes in the U.S. contains dangerous levels of radon gas. Radon gas is invisible and odorless, but can be detected with simple test kits.

Lung disease

The presence of certain diseases of the lung, notably chronic obstructive pulmonary disease (COPD), is associated with a slightly increased risk (four to six times the risk of a nonsmoker) for the development of lung cancer even after the effects of concomitant cigarette smoking are excluded.

Prior history of lung cancer

Survivors of lung cancer have a greater risk than the general population of developing a second lung cancer. Survivors of non-small cell lung cancers have an added risk of 1%-2% per year for developing a second lung cancer. In survivors of small cell lung cancers, the risk for development of second cancers approaches 6% per year.

Air pollution

Air pollution from vehicles, industry, and power plants, can raise the likelihood of developing lung cancer. Up to 1% of lung cancer deaths are attributable to breathing polluted air, and experts believe that prolonged exposure to highly polluted air can carry a risk similar to that of passive smoking for the development of lung cancer.

Genetic

While the majority of lung cancers are associated with tobacco smoking, the fact that not all smokers eventually develop lung cancer suggests that other factors, such as individual genetic susceptibility, may play a role in the causation of lung cancer. Numerous studies have shown that lung cancer is more likely to occur in both smoking and nonsmoking relatives of those who have had lung cancer than in the general population.

Types of Lung Cancer

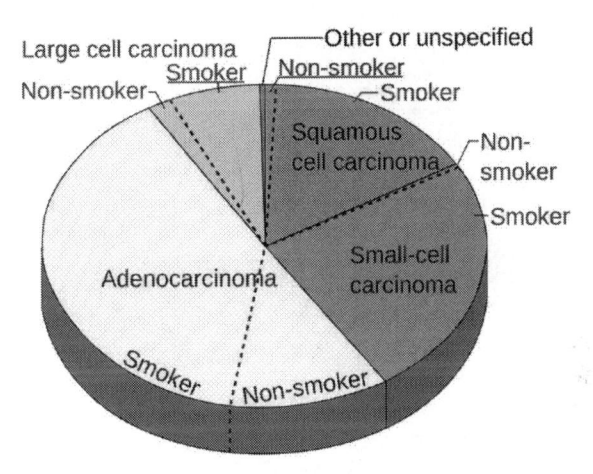

Lung cancers are broadly classified into two types: small cell lung cancers (SCLC) and non-small cell lung cancers (NSCLC). This classification is based upon the microscopic appearance of the tumor cells. These two types of cancers grow, spread, and treated in different ways, so making a distinction between these two types is important.

Small cell lung cancers (SCLC)

SCLC comprises about 10%-15% of lung cancers. This type of lung cancer is the most aggressive and rapidly growing of all the types. SCLC is strongly related to cigarette smoking. SCLCs metastasize rapidly to many sites within the body and are most often discovered after they have spread extensively.

Non-small cell lung cancers (NSCLC)

NSCLC is the most common lung cancer, accounting for about 85% of all cases. NSCLC has three main types designated by the type of cells found in the tumor. They are:

Adenocarcinoma

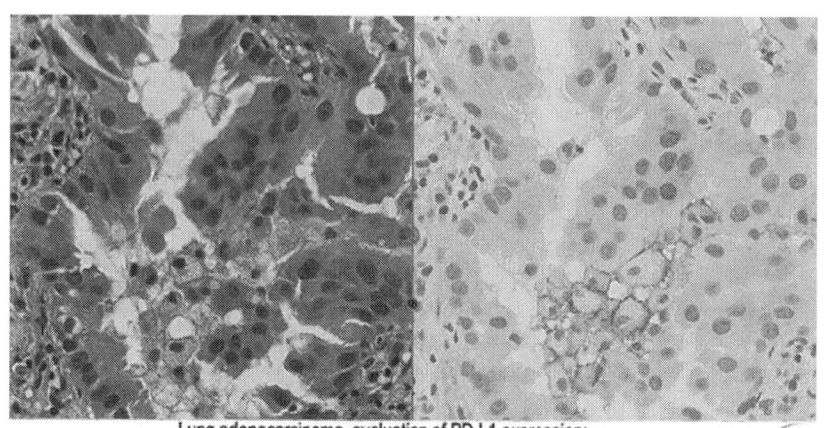

Lung adenocarcinoma, evaluation of PD-L1 expression: membranous staining in macrophages, all cancer cells are negative for anti-PD-L1, score 0 (×40)

Adenocarcinomas are the most common type of NSCLC in the U.S. and comprise up to 40% of lung cancer cases. While adenocarcinomas are associated with smoking like other lung cancers, this type is also seen in non-smokers - especially women - who develop lung cancer. Most adenocarcinomas arise in the outer, or peripheral, areas of the lungs. They also have a tendency to spread to the lymph nodes and beyond. Adenocarcinoma in situ (previously called bronchioloalveolar carcinoma) is a subtype of adenocarcinoma that frequently develops at multiple sites in the lungs and spreads along the pre-existing alveolar walls. It may also look like pneumonia on a chest X-ray. It is increasing in frequency and is more common in women. People with this type of lung cancer tend to have a better prognosis than those with other types of lung cancer.

Squamous cell carcinomas

Squamous cell carcinomas were formerly more common than adenocarcinomas; today, they account for about 25% to 30% of all lung cancer cases. Also known as epidermoid carcinomas, squamous cell cancers arise most frequently in the central chest area in the bronchi. This type of lung cancer, most often stays within the lung, spreads to lymph nodes, and grows quite large, forming a cavity.

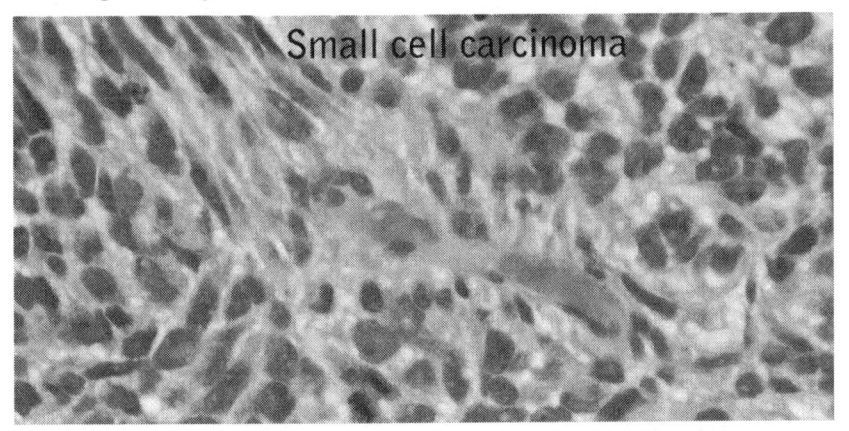

Large cell carcinomas

Large cell carcinomas, sometimes referred to as undifferentiated carcinomas, are the least common type of NSCLC, accounting for 10%-15% of all lung cancers. This type of cancer has a high tendency to spread to the lymph nodes and distant sites.

Other types of cancers can arise in the lung; these types are much less common than NSCLC and SCLC and together comprise only 5%-10% of lung cancers:

- Bronchial carcinoids account for up to 5% of lung cancers. These tumors are generally small (3-4 cm or less) when diagnosed and occur most commonly in persons under age 40. Unrelated to cigarette smoking, carcinoid tumors can metastasize, and a small proportion of these tumors secrete hormone-like substances. Carcinoids generally grow and spread more slowly than bronchogenic cancers, and many are detected early enough to be surgically removed.
- Cancers of supporting lung tissue such as smooth muscle, blood vessels, or cells involved in the immune response are rare in the lung.

- Metastatic cancers from other primary tumors in the body are often found in the lung. Tumors from anywhere in the body may spread to the lungs either through the bloodstream, through the lymphatic system, or directly from nearby organs. Metastatic tumors are most often multiple, scattered throughout the lung and concentrated in the outer areas rather than central areas of the organ.

Symptoms and signs

There are various types of symptoms in this disease, which depend on tumors size, location and metastasis. There are generally no obvious and serious symptoms of cancer in the early stages.

No Symptoms

25% of lung cancer patients are diagnosed with X-ray or CT scan done for routine testing or investigations done for other purpose. Often, a coin shaped shadow in the x-ray produces suspicion of cancer. Often these patients do not have any symptoms.

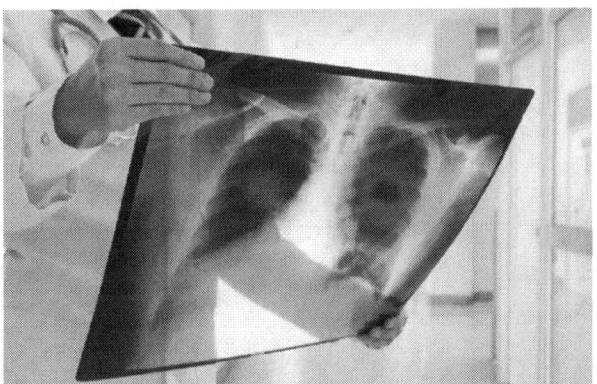

Symptoms related to the cancer:

- Patient feels **difficulty in breathing** due to the tumor and its spread in the lungs.
- A cough that does not go away or gets worse
- Coughing up blood or rust-colored sputum (spit or phlegm)

- Chest pain that is often worse with deep breathing, coughing, or laughing
- Hoarseness
- Weight loss and loss of appetite
- Shortness of breath
- Feeling tired or weak
- Infections such as bronchitis and pneumonia that don't go away or keep coming back
- New onset of wheezing

Symptoms related to metastasis:

- Bone pain (like pain in the back or hips)
- Nervous system changes (such as headache, weakness or numbness of an arm or leg, dizziness, balance problems, or seizures), from cancer spread to the brain or spinal cord
- Yellow coloration of the skin and eyes (jaundice), from cancer spread to the liver
- Lumps near the surface of the body, due to cancer spreading to the skin or to lymph nodes (collections of immune system cells), such as those in the neck or above the collarbone
- Most of these symptoms are more likely to be caused by something other than lung cancer. Still, if you have any of these problems, it's important to see your doctor right away so the cause can be found and treated, if needed.

Some lung cancers can cause Syndromes, which are groups of very specific symptoms.

Horner syndrome

Cancers of the top part of the lungs (sometimes called Pancoast tumors) sometimes can affect certain nerves to the eye

and part of the face, causing a group of symptoms called Horner syndrome:
- Drooping or weakness of one eyelid
- A smaller pupil (dark part in the center of the eye) in the same eye
- Reduced or absent sweating on the same side of the face
- Pancoast tumors can also sometimes cause severe shoulder pain.

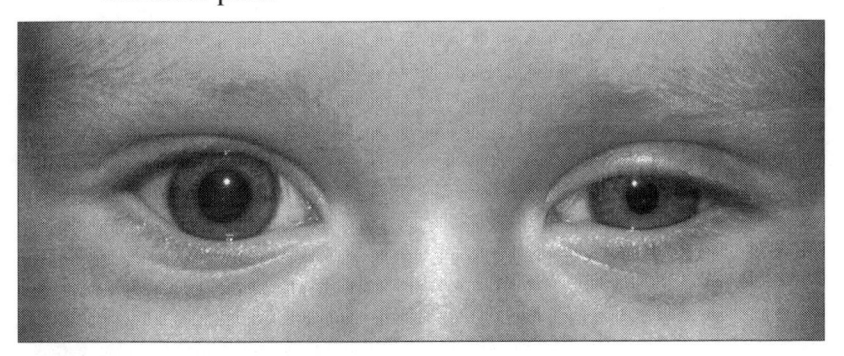

Superior vena cava syndrome

The superior vena cava (SVC) is a large vein that carries blood from the head and arms back to the heart. It passes next to the upper part of the right lung and the lymph nodes inside the chest. Tumors in this area can press on the SVC, which can cause the blood to back up in the veins. This can lead to swelling in the face, neck, arms, and upper chest (sometimes with a bluish-red skin color). It can also cause headaches, dizziness, and a change in consciousness if it affects the brain. While SVC syndrome can develop gradually over time, in some cases it can become life-threatening, and needs to be treated right away.

Paraneoplastic syndromes

Some lung cancers can make hormone-like substances that enter the bloodstream and cause problems with distant tissues and organs, even though the cancer has not spread to those tissues or organs. These problems are called paraneoplastic syndromes.

Sometimes these syndromes can be the first symptoms of lung cancer. Because the symptoms affect organs other than the lungs, patients and their doctors may suspect at first that a disease other than lung cancer is causing them.

Some of the more common paraneoplastic syndromes associated with lung cancer are:
- **SIADH** (syndrome of inappropriate anti-diuretic hormone): In this condition, the cancer cells make a hormone (ADH) that causes the kidneys to retain water. This lowers salt levels in the blood. Symptoms of SIADH can include fatigue, loss of appetite, muscle weakness or cramps, nausea, vomiting, restlessness, and confusion. Without treatment, severe cases may lead to seizures and coma.
- **Cushing syndrome:** In this condition, the cancer cells may make ACTH, a hormone that causes the adrenal glands to secrete cortisol. This can lead to symptoms such as weight gain, easy bruising, weakness, drowsiness, and fluid retention. Cushing syndrome can also cause high blood pressure and high blood sugar levels (or even diabetes).
- **Nervous system problems:** Lung cancer can sometimes cause the body's immune system to attack parts of the nervous system, which can lead to problems. One example is a muscle disorder called the Lambert-Eaton syndrome, in which the muscles around the hips become weak. One of the first signs may be trouble getting up from a sitting position. Later, muscles around the shoulder may become weak. A rarer problem is paraneoplastic cerebellar degeneration, which can cause loss of balance and unsteadiness in arm and leg movement, as well as trouble speaking or swallowing.
- **High blood calcium levels (hypercalcemia):** This can cause frequent urination, thirst, constipation, nausea, vomiting, belly pain, weakness, fatigue, dizziness, confusion, and other nervous system problems

- Excess growth or thickening of certain bones: This is often in the finger tips, and can be painful.
- Blood clots
- Excess breast growth in men (gynecomastia)

Again, many of these symptoms are more likely to be caused by something other than lung cancer. Still, if you have any of these problems, it's important to see your doctor right away so the cause can be found and treated, if needed.

When should you consult the doctor?

If the patient has the following symptoms, then contact the doctor immediately:
- Fast cough or chronic cough may suddenly increase
- Coughing in cough
- Pain in chest
- Acute bronchitis or frequent respiratory tract infection
- Sudden weight loss or fatigue occurs
- Disinfection or wheezing occurs

Diagnostic Workup

History and clinical examination

In the inquiry and examination of the patient, the doctor often finds some symptoms and signs that point to the cancer. He asks about smoking history, cough, any shortness of breath, any obstruction in respiratory tract, infection etc. Bluish coloration of skin or mucus indicates lack of oxygen in the blood (Cyanosis). The clubbing of nails reflects chronic lung disease.

Chest X-ray

A chest x-ray is usually the first test performed to evaluate any concerns based on a careful history and physical. This may show a mass in the lungs or enlarged lymph nodes. Sometimes the chest x-ray is normal, and further tests are needed look for a suspected lung cancer. It should be stressed that a chest x-ray alone is not sufficient to rule out lung cancer, and early cancers can easily be missed with these tests.

Though the shadow visible in the lung X-ray creates suspicion of cancer. But X-ray does not prove that this shadow is of cancer itself, calcified nodules or a benign tumors also cast a similar shadow in the lungs. Therefore, other tests are done to confirm the diagnosis.

CT scan (computerized tomography)

Usually chest, abdomen, and brain C.T. scan is performed to diagnose lung cancer and metastatic cancer. A CT scan is frequently the second step either to follow up on an abnormal chest x-ray finding or to evaluate troublesome symptoms in those with a normal chest x-ray. A CT scan uses x-rays to make detailed cross-sectional images of your body. Instead of taking one picture, like a regular x-ray, a CT scanner takes many pictures as it rotates around you while you lie on a table. This data is transmitted to a computer, which builds up a 3-D cross-sectional picture of the part of the body and displays it on the screen. Sometimes, a contrast dye is used because it can help show certain structures more clearly. Sensitivity test is done before giving contrast injection. Many times it can cause symptoms of harmful reaction such as itching, skin rashes etc. or deadly anaphylactic reaction in rare patients. CT scans are more precise to show lung tumors than routine chest x-rays. They can also show the size, shape, and position of any lung tumor and can help find enlarged lymph nodes that might contain cancer that has spread from the lung. C.T. scan of abdomen also detects metastatic cancer of liver and adrenal glands. C.T. scan of brain detects brain's metastatic cancer.

MRI (Magnetic resonance imaging)

For clear and detailed images of the tumor, MRI is considered more suitable. MRI takes images of body parts with the help of magnet, radio waves and computer. Just like CT scan, the patient is laid on a motorized table and passed through the machine. There is no side-effect and there is no danger of radiation. The images are more elaborate and it also captures very small nodules. If the patient's heart has prosthetic valves, pacemaker, or metal implant in the body, then the MRI should not be done because it can damage these devices.

Positron emission tomography (PET scanning)

This is the most sensitive, specific and expensive investigation. In this, fluorinated glucose (18 FDG) such as radioactive labeled metabolite is used, and accurate, detailed, multicolored and three-dimensional pictures and information about tumor metabolism, vascularisation, oxygen consumption and tissue receptor status is collected, processed and displayed on a monitor screen. C.T. scan and MRI gives us only the structure of the tumor, while PET scan gives information about the tissue's metabolic activity and functioning. PET scan also gives information about the growth of the tumor and also explains what types of cancer cells the tumor is made of.

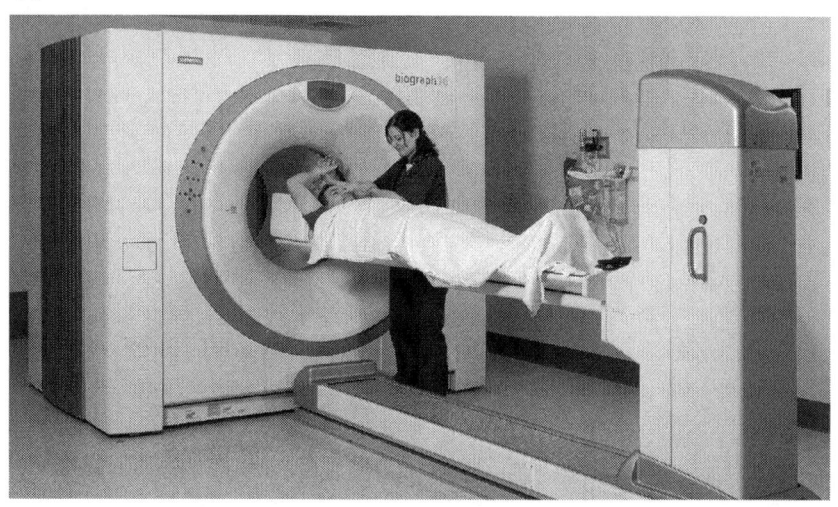

A short half-lived radioactive drug is given to the patient, and a small dose of radiation is given as two chest x-rays. This drug is more concentrated in certain tissues (like cancer) than other tissues of the body, depending on the given medication. With the effect of radiation, this drug discharges the particle called positron, which encounters with the electrons in the body from. This reaction produces gamma rays. A scanner records these gamma rays and maps the area where the radioactive drug has accumulated. For example, the radioactive drug found in glucose (the source of normal energy) would tell which tissues consumed glucose rapidly, such as developing and active tumor cells. PET scanning may also be integrated with CT scanning in a technique known as PET-CT scanning. This technique determines the stage of cancer PET and proved to be a boon in cancer diagnosis.

Bone scan

Pictures of bones are taken on the screen or film of the computer by the bone scan. Doctor bone scans do this to know that lung cancer has not reached bones. For this, a radioactive medicine is released in the patient's vein. This drug is collected in the bones at that place where metastasis cancer has taken place. The machine's scanner accepts radioactive medicine and takes a picture of the affected bone on the film.

Bone scans are used to create images of bones on a computer screen or on film. Doctors may order a bone scan to determine whether a lung cancer has metastasized to the bones. In a bone scan, a small amount of radioactive material is injected into the bloodstream and collects in the bones, especially in abnormal areas such as those involved by metastatic tumors. The radioactive material is detected by a scanner, and the image of the bones is recorded on a special film for permanent viewing.

Sputum cytology

Sputum cytology is a quick and inexpensive test; however, it is not always accurate. Sputum cytology is the testing of lung secretions or phlegm to look for cancer cells. The patient coughs up a sample of mucus, which is viewed under the microscope to identify possible cancer cells. Samples are often collected early in the morning for several days. Sputum cytology is more useful in diagnosing squamous cell lung cancers, which start in the central airways, and may not be as effective in identifying other types of lung cancer, particularly those located in more distant areas of the lungs. Sputum cytology detects approximately 71% of tumors that are centrally located, but it detects less than 50% of tumors that are located in the periphery (outer regions) of the lungs.

When the results are positive for cancer, sputum cytology does not provide enough information for doctors to be able to determine exactly what type of lung cancer a patient has. A biopsy is required to get a good sample of the tumor and identify the type of lung cancer.

Bronchoscopy

Bronchoscopy is a test that allows a doctor to view the airways (bronchi) with the use of a thin, lighted tube containing a camera. The tube used in bronchoscopy may be flexible or rigid. The flexible scope is most often used. The rigid scope is a straight tube and is only used to view the larger airways. Bronchoscopy, also called fiberoptic bronchoscopy, is used to diagnose and sometimes treat lung conditions. If lung cancer is suspected, bronchoscopy can provide a way for the doctor to view the tumor, assess the extent of the airway obstruction (blockage), and collect a tissue sample for biopsy. Bronchoscopy is most often used for diagnosing lung cancer when the suspicious lesion is centrally located, rather than those that are in the periphery, or distant regions of the lungs.

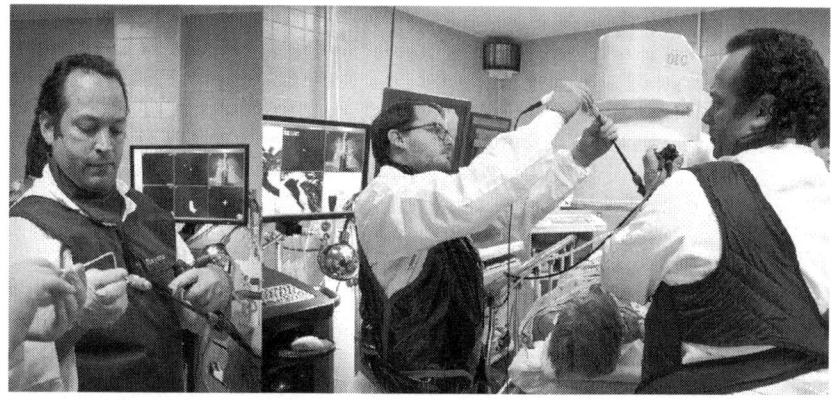

Patients are often advised not to eat or drink anything for 6-12 hours prior to having a bronchoscopy. Additional instructions are provided by the doctor and may include stopping the use of some medications, such as aspirin, ibuprofen or other drugs that may increase bleeding risk. Usually, the test is done as an outpatient procedure, meaning the patient does not need to stay in the hospital overnight. The patient is given anesthetic to relax and numb the throat muscles. The tube-like instrument, the bronchoscope, is placed through the nose or mouth and guided down into the airways of the lungs. The camera at the end of the tube displays images back to a video screen.

Bronchoscopy is generally a safe procedure, but it should be performed by experienced doctor. After the anesthetic wears off, the patient may experience a scratchy throat for several days.

Serious complications are uncommon (less than 5% of patients), such as an air leak or serious bleeding. Possible side effects from a bronchoscopy include reduced oxygen, lung leak or collapse, bleeding from biopsy sites, infection, arrhythmias (abnormal cardiac rhythms), difficulty in breathing, fever, or a heart attack in people with existing heart disease.

Fine needle aspiration Cytology (FNAC)

This is the most common test in which a needle is inserted into the cancerous growth in the lungs with the guidance of CT scan, and samples of cells are taken for microscopy. If the cancerous tumor is located in the outer parts of the lungs and where the bronchoscope does not reach, then this technique is very useful. With lung cancer, the needle is inserted into the chest through the skin on the chest and into a tumor which is often found on a CT scan of the chest. Doctors can make sure the needle goes to the right part of the lung by watching it through ultrasound or a CT scanner, and then the cells are aspirated by putting syringe in the needle. But sometimes the doctor does not succeed in taking tissues from the right place. This technique has a risk of having pneumothorax.

Thoracentesis

Thoracentesis is a procedure in which a needle or small tube is used to remove excess fluid in the pleural space, the space between the lungs and the chest wall. Fluid can build up as a result of lung cancer, as well as from other conditions like infections, injury, heart or liver failure, or blood clots in the lungs. This fluid build-up is called pleural effusion, and while some people experience no symptoms with pleural effusion, others experience chest pain that may worsen with deep breathing or coughing, dry cough, shortness of breath, difficulty in breathing, rapid breathing, fever, or hiccups. When fluid occupies the pleural space, the lungs do not have space to properly inflate. Removing the fluid helps the patient to breathe easier.

Thoracentesis can be used both to remove the fluid and determine the cause of the fluid build-up. After the fluid is removed, a laboratory may examine the fluid. Thoracentesis can be one of the procedures used to assist a physician in diagnosing lung cancer. There is also little risk of pneumothorax in this technique.

Major surgical procedure

If cancer cannot be diagnosed with all the above methods, then surgery remains the last option. The first option is mediastinoscopy, in which samples of cells are taken from the tumor or lymph node by surgically inserting a probe between the two lungs. The second option is thoracotomy, in which the tissue samples are taken by opening the chest. It is not possible to remove the tumor completely by these surgeries. For this, the patient is admitted and the surgery is performed only in the operation theater. Also there is risk of bleeding, infection, anesthesia and side effects of the medicines.

Laboratory Tests

There are several laboratory tests that may be done during the diagnosis and staging of lung cancer. Laboratory tests are any procedure that evaluates a sample of blood, urine, other bodily fluid, or tissue. Some tests provide specific information about a condition, while others rule out other problems (determine other problems don't exist) or provide general information about the patient's overall health and chemical or metabolic disorders caused by cancer.

While there is not a single laboratory test that can determine if a person has lung cancer (confirmation of lung cancer occurs after lung cells are examined through a microscope), the tests can provide additional information that helps doctors determine the best course of treatment for the individual.

Complete Blood Count (CBC)

A complete blood count is a test that measures all the different components in the blood. Blood contains several different cells: red blood cells, white blood cells, and platelets. The complete blood count measures the levels of these cells, as well as the levels of hemoglobin (an iron-rich protein in red blood cells that carries oxygen), hematocrit (a percentage representing the space that red blood cells occupy in the blood) reticulocyte count (a percentage representing the number of young red blood cells in the blood), and mean corpuscular volume (the average size of red blood cells).

Some of the abnormal findings from a CBC include:
- Low levels of red blood cells can indicate anemia
- Low levels of blood platelets can point to a tendency to bleed and difficulty forming clots
- Low levels of white blood cells can place a person at higher risk for infections

In addition to doing a CBC during diagnosis, CBC is often done during chemotherapy courses to monitor side effects of treatments.

Blood Chemistry Tests

Blood chemistry tests detect various levels of substances in the body and can identify abnormalities in some of the organs. If lung cancer has spread, it can change the functional ability of the organ in which it spreads to, creating an imbalance in the levels of markers found in the blood, such as electrolytes, metabolites, fats, and proteins, including enzymes.

If the level of calcium and enzyme alkaline phosphatase increases, indicates cancer metastasis in the bone. Similarly, aspirate aminotransferase (SGOT) and alanine aminotransferase (SGPT) increases the liver disorder, probably due to which the

liver should have metastatic cancer. Following tests should be performed to diagnose liver metastatic disease.
- CBC
- Electrolytes
- Parathyroid hormone
- Aspartate aminotransferase (SGOT), alanine aminotransferase (SGPT), alkaline phosphatease, prothrombin time

Molecular Profiling (Genetic Testing)

One of the most exciting advances in the treatment of lung cancer has come from an understanding of genetic changes in lung cancer cells. Whereas in the past we classified lung cancers down into perhaps five types, we now know that no two lung cancers are the same. If there were 30 people in a room with lung cancer, they would have 30 different and unique types of the disease.

If you've been recently diagnosed with lung cancer, especially lung adenocarcinoma, your oncologist may have talked to you about genetic testing (otherwise known as molecular profiling or biomarker testing) of your tumor. It's now recommended that all lung cancer patients with advanced or metastatic lung adenocarcinoma (a type of non-small cell lung cancer) have biomarker testing to look for EGFR mutations and ALK and ROS1 rearrangements.

In addition, patients with other forms of non-small cell lung cancer (for example, squamous cell carcinoma in non-smokers) should also be considered for testing.

Genetic Testing

Genetic testing involves tests that a pathologist performs in a lab using a sample of your cancer tissue. These tests look at cancer from a molecular level.

The tissue may come from a biopsy of your tumor or from tissue removed during surgery for lung cancer. The reason behind this is that cancers have gene mutations and other changes that "drive" or control the growth of cancer.

Simplistically, if these mutations can be identified, then treatments can be used which "target" these mutations, hence stopping the growth of cancer. It is these mutations that lead to the development of cancer in the first place.

Before going further, it's helpful to address something that is confusing for many people. There are two primary types of gene mutations:

Hereditary mutations - Also called germline mutations, this means you inherit genes with mutations from one or more parents. Common examples of these mutations include hemophilia as well as mutations that may predispose someone to developing breast cancer, like BRCA1 and BRCA2.

Acquired mutations - The type of mutations that scientists actually look for in people with lung cancer is called acquired mutations or somatic mutation). These mutations are not present at birth (and do not run in families), but rather develop in the process of cells becoming cancerous.

What Are Gene Mutations?

Gene mutations are changes to a particular gene in a chromosome. All genes are made up of variable sequences of four amino acids (called bases)—adenine, tyrosine, cytosine, and guanine.

When a gene is exposed to toxins in the environment, or when an accident occurs in cell division, a mutation, or change, may occur. In some cases, it may mean that one base is substituted for another, like adenine instead of guanine. In other cases, bases may be inserted, deleted, or rearranged in some way.

Significance of Gene Mutations

Why are oncologists interested in acquired gene mutations in a tumor? First, we should talk about the two types of acquired mutations found in lung cancers:

Driver mutations - These mutations, via several mechanisms, "drive" the growth of a tumor. In lung cancer, the number of driver mutations is variable. In one study, an average of 11 driver mutations per cancer was found.

Passenger mutations - Just as someone may be a passenger in a car, these genes do not drive cancer, but are basically along for the ride. Again, we don't know exactly how many passenger mutations are present in a tumor (and the number varies from tumor to tumor), but some tumors may have more than 1,000 of these mutations. Driver mutations not only initiate the development of cancer, but work to maintain the growth of cancer as well.

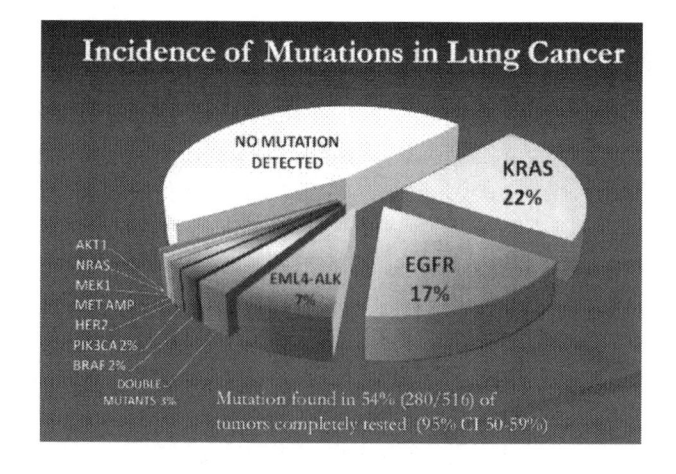

Incidence of Mutations in Lung Cancer

- NO MUTATION DETECTED
- KRAS 22%
- EGFR 17%
- EML4-ALK 7%
- AKT1
- NRAS
- MEK1
- MET AMP
- HER2
- PIK3CA 2%
- BRAF 2%
- DOUBLE MUTANTS 3%

Mutation found in 54% (280/516) of tumors completely tested (95% CI 50-59%)

Common Driver Mutations

There are many mutations that are being studied by scientists looking at lung tumors. So far, driver mutations have been identified in approximately 60 percent of lung adenocarcinomas and it's likely this number will increase in time.

Researchers are now finding driver mutations in squamous cell lung cancer as well. In general, these mutations are mutually exclusive and are only rarely seen in the same tumor. Common driver mutations in lung cancer include:

- EGFR mutations
- KRAS mutations
- EML4-ALK rearrangements
- ROS1 rearrangements
- MET amplifications
- HER2 mutations
- RET rearrangements
- BRAF mutations

Personalized Treatments

The use of "targeted therapies," medications that target particular genetic abnormalities in a tumor, has been coined personalized medicine or precision medicine. What this means is that, rather than a conventional chemotherapy drug that attacks all rapidly dividing cells, a targeted drug attacks a particular abnormality present only in your cancer cells.

In general, targeted treatments have fewer side effects than traditional chemotherapy. To date, targeted therapies that have been approved for people with lung cancer include:

Tarceva (erlotinib) for people whose tumor has an EGFR mutation (Note: there are different types of EGFR mutations and not all of them are equally responsive to this.)

Xalkori (crizotinib) for people whose tumor has an EML4-ALK gene rearrangement. The FDA approved this in 2011 and it then was granted breakthrough status for ROS1 rearranged lung cancer in 2015.

Other medications have been approved and are being studied in clinical trials, including targeted therapies for those whose tumor becomes resistant to Tarceva or Xalkori.

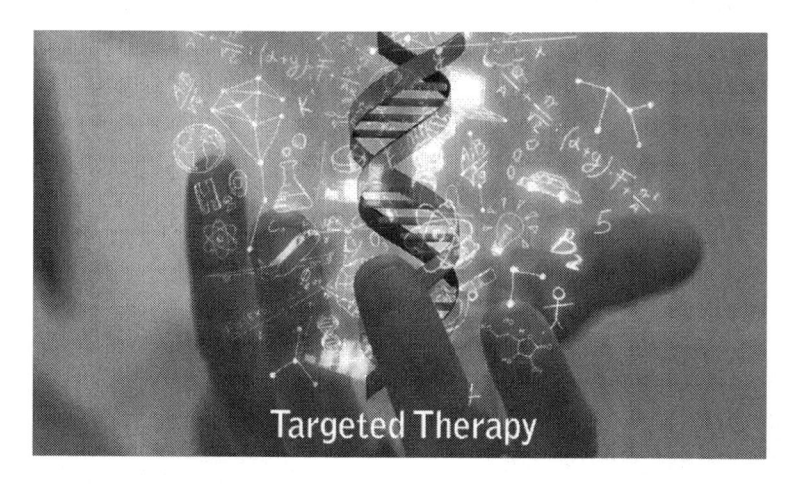

Resistance to Treatment

A challenging problem with currently used targeted treatments is that nearly everyone inevitably becomes resistant to treatments we have. There are many mechanisms by which this occurs making it difficult to find one solution. Research is ongoing in clinical trials—evaluating both the use of substituting a second drug to target the mutations and drugs that use different targets or mechanisms to attack the cancer cell.

Testing

Testing for gene mutations and rearrangements is usually performed on tissue samples obtained from some form of lung biopsy or biopsy of a metastasis. As of June 2016, however, a liquid biopsy test is now available as a method of testing for EGFR mutations in some people. Since these tests can be done with a simple blood draw, this is an exciting advance in monitoring lung cancer.

A Word from "Very well Health"

The ability to understand the molecular profile of lung tumors is an extremely exciting area of research, and it's likely that new treatments for other mutations will soon be available.

An example of how rapidly this area of medicine is advancing is the EML4-ALK gene rearrangement. This gene "mutation" (actually a rearrangement) was discovered as recently as 2007. Through a rapid process, the medication Xalkori (crizotinib) was approved in 2011 for general use by the FDA for those patients whose tumors have this rearrangement. There are clinical trials currently in progress evaluating the use of second-generation drugs for those who have become resistant to Xalkori.

If you have been diagnosed with non-small cell lung cancer, especially lung adenocarcinoma or squamous cell lung cancer, talk to your doctor about genetic testing. Although testing is now recommended for everyone with advanced non-small cell lung cancer, a recent study reported that only 60 percent of oncologists are currently ordering testing.

You may also wish to talk to your doctor about clinical trials that may be an option for you. Recently, a lung cancer clinical trial matching service backed by several lung cancer organizations has become available, too. With this free service, a trained nurse navigator can help you locate any clinical trials that may be an option for you.

Tumor markers in lung cancer

Blood tumor markers may warn when lung cancer patients are progressing. For many years, oncologists have known that cancers can secrete complex molecules into the blood and that levels of these molecules can be easily measured. These so-called 'tumor markers' are traditionally associated with a single dominant cancer type, for example Prostate Specific Antigen (PSA) linked to prostate cancer, Carcinoembryonic antigen (CEA) to colorectal cancer, CA125 to ovarian cancer, CA19.9 to pancreatic cancer and CA27.29 to breast cancer. However, the real challenge has been to determine a practical use for these markers. They don't appear to be useful as a means of screening otherwise healthy people for evidence of underlying cancers.

Now a University of Colorado Cancer Center has begun study to further define the potential of these markers by looking in a type of cancer not normally associated with them - non-small cell lung cancer (NSCLC). The study suggests that rather than screening for disease, these tumor markers could be useful in monitoring therapeutic outcomes in those with already established disease.

"If you ask some oncologists they might say that there's no point checking these markers in lung cancer as it don't express them," says D. Ross Camidge, MD, PhD, Joyce Zeff Chair in Lung Cancer Research at the University of Colorado Cancer Center and director of Thoracic Oncology at the CU School of Medicine. However, when Camidge and colleagues examined levels of four markers classically associated with other cancers, namely CEA, CA125, CA19.9 and CA27.29, they found that if all four were checked, at least one of them was elevated in 95 percent of advanced non-small cell lung cancers (NSCLCs). Some cases expressed only one marker; others expressed multiple markers together.

In recent years, dramatic anti-cancer responses have become possible for some patients with advanced NSCLC with targeted therapies used against specific mutations. By focusing on some of the most prominent examples of 'oncogene-addicted' NSCLC - notably, cases of advanced EGFR, ALK or ROS1 positive NSCLC treated with the appropriate EGFR, ALK or ROS1 targeted therapy - the Colorado group was able to study the potential for these blood tumor markers to reflect both initial therapeutic outcomes and the later development of treatment resistance.

In 126 patients with stage IV oncogene-addicted lung cancer, tumor markers were captured before and after the initiation of treatment. Among patients on targeted treatment expected to have a high response rate, 59 percent of patients had an initial increase in their marker levels during the first four weeks of therapy, with the elevated levels later falling below baseline values in 58 percent of cases.

"These data mean that you shouldn't worry about marker elevations in the first few weeks of targeted therapy in the absence of other evidence, such as worsening symptoms, as most of the time things settle down. Perhaps tumor markers shouldn't even be checked during this early time period at all," Camidge says.

While the tumor markers may not be very useful for predicting initial success or failure, once a patient is benefiting from a targeted treatment, increases in tumor markers from their lowest point may provide useful information about the development of resistance. When a patient's cancer was progressing in the body, a 10 percent or greater rise in the blood tumor markers occurred in 53 percent of patients. However, if the progression was limited to the brain, the tumor markers went up in only 22 percent of cases.

"Clearly, these markers are not a substitute for routine surveillance scans looking for progression, especially in the brain," says Camidge. "However, this is where the art of medicine may have to be appreciated. If the markers are going up but a CT scan says everything is still fine, maybe these data should nudge you to do a more detailed scan - like a PET/CT scan. Or if the best body scans are all stable, perhaps a rise in tumor markers should nudge you to do a brain scan looking harder for a hidden site of progression."

Despite patients in this retrospective study having undergone multiple different types of scans and blood draws at many different frequencies, the data still show that rises in tumor markers on therapy could occur well in advance of radiographic changes of progression (up to 84 days). Although Camidge says a prospective, randomized trial is needed to fully validate the potential of these markers to act as an early warning system, the real question may turn out to be whether finding progression several months' earlier matters.

"If adapting your treatment plan earlier versus later in progression doesn't impact outcomes, an early warning system could just give everyone more time to stress about things," he says. However, particularly for oncogene-addicted lung cancer, in which national guidelines now support using strategies such as targeted radiation to control small pockets of treatment-resistant disease, Camidge is optimistic that an early warning system for progression could be very useful.

"An 'oligoprogressive' state gives us therapeutic options that we wouldn't have if the progression was more widespread," he says. "Developing means to catch this earlier 'stage' of progression in more people should definitely be explored further."

Staging

If you're trying to figure out the stage of your lung cancer you might be feeling very confused. What does it mean when your oncologist talks about "TNM" and how is this correlated with the stages? Let's take a look at the meaning of each of these letters, how doctors use these to stage a cancer, and what that ultimately means in terms of treatment.

The TNM System

TNM staging for lung cancer can be confusing for anyone to understand, let alone someone who has just been hit with the news of a lung cancer diagnosis. How does TNM staging align with the lung cancer stages, like stage 2 and stage 4? The TNM system is used for all lung carcinomas except SCLCs.

What the Letters Mean

Each of the TNM letters stands for the size or spread of a cancer as follows:

- **T** – Stands for the size of the tumor. Tumor size is usually given in centimeters (cm). To understand this in inches, 5 cm is about the same as 2 inches.
- **N** – N stands for lymph nodes and tells whether the tumor has spread to lymph nodes, and if so, how far away from the tumor they are.
- **M** – M stands for metastasis, that is, the spread of the tumor to other parts of the body.

Why Staging Is Important

TNM staging helps doctors understand how extensive a cancer is and, therefore, what the best treatment options are for that particular cancer. It can also help predict what the average prognosis is for someone with lung cancer. TNM staging is based on worldwide data on lung cancer in thousands of people and compares of the extent of lung cancer with responses to treatment and prognosis.

That said it is very important to understand that there are many factors that affect the prognosis of lung cancer that go beyond the stage. Your general health, the particular type of lung cancer you have, whether or not you have "targetable" gene mutations in your tumor, and even your gender can play a role in what treatments will work best for you and what your individual prognosis may be.

TNM Staging

You will notice that your TNM letters will have numbers which follow them. Let's look at what the different numbers mean:

T - Tumor Size

- **Tx** – The tumor size is unknown, or cancer cells are only found in sputum.
- **T0** – There is no evidence of a primary tumor.
- **Tis** – Carcinoma in situ – The tumor is present only in the cells lining the airway and has not spread to nearby tissues.
- **T1** – Tumors less than or equal to 3 cm (1 ½ inches).
    - T1a – Less than or equal to 2 cm.
    - T1b – Greater than 2 cm but less than or equal to 3 cm.
- T2 – The tumor is greater than 3 cm but less than 7 cm. T2 tumors may block part of the airway, but have not resulted in pneumonia or caused the lung to collapse (atelectasis). They may have spread to the lining around the lungs. They may also be close to the main bronchus

but are at least 2 cm (about an inch) away from the area in which the bronchus divides to go to each of the lungs.
- T2a – Greater than 3 cm but less than or equal to 5 cm.
- T2b – Greater than 5 cm but less than or equal to 7 cm.

- **T3** – Tumors greater than 7 cm, or less than 7 cm but with a separate nodule in the same lobe. T3 tumors also include tumors that are less than 7 cm but invade the lining of the lung (pleura), the chest wall, the diaphragm, the main bronchus, or lie within 2 cm of the area where the bronchus divides to travel to the lungs. A tumor is also classified as T3 if it is less than 7 cm but is associated with pneumonia or collapse of the entire lung.

- **T4** – A tumor of any size, but with another nodule in a different lobe on the same side of the body, or a tumor that invades structures in the chest such as the heart, major blood vessels near the heart, the trachea, the recurrent laryngeal nerve (a nerve near the trachea), the mediastinum (the space between the lungs), the esophagus, or the area where the main bronchus divides to travel to the two lungs.

N – Involvement of Lymph Nodes
- **N0** – No nodes are involved.
- **N1**   The tumor has spread to nearby nodes on the same side of the body.
- **N2** – The tumor has spread to nodes farther away but on the same side of the chest.

- **N3** – The tumor has spread to lymph nodes on the other side of the chest from the original tumor, or has spread to nodes near the collarbone or neck muscles.

M – Metastasis (Spread) to Other Regions
- **M0** - The tumor has not spread to distant regions.
- **M1**
    - **M1a** – The tumor has spread to the opposite lung, to the lung lining (malignant pleural effusion) or has formed nodules on the pleura.
    - **M1b** – The tumor has spread to distant regions of the body, such as the brain or bones.

Comparison of Lung Cancer Stages and TNM Staging

Most people are more familiar with the stages of lung cancer than they are with TNM staging. Here is a comparison of lung cancer stages and TNM staging:

Stage 0 Lung Cancer
- TisN0M0

Stage 1 Lung Cancer
- **Stage 1A Lung Cancer**
    - T1aN0M0
    - T1bN0M0

- **Stage 1B Lung Cancer**
    - T2aN0M0

Stage 2 Lung Cancer
- **Stage 2A Lung Cancer**

- T1aN1M0
- T1bN0M0
- T2aN1M0
- **Stage 2B Lung Cancer**
    - T2bN0M0
    - T2bN1M0
    - T3N0M0

Stage 3 Lung Cancer
- **Stage 3A Lung Cancer**
    - T3N1M0
    - T4N0M0
    - T4N1M0
    - T1N2M0
    - T2N2M0
    - T3N2M0
- **Stage 3B Lung Cancer**
    - T1N3M0
    - T2N3M0
    - T3N3M0
    - T4N2M0
    - T4N3M0

- **Stage 4 Lung Cancer**
    - Any T, Any N, M1a
    - Any T, Any N, M1b

Treatment

Lung cancer is treated in several ways, depending on the type of lung cancer and how far it has spread. People with non-small cell lung cancer can be treated with surgery, chemotherapy, radiation therapy, targeted therapy, or a combination of these treatments. People with small cell lung cancer are usually treated with radiation therapy and chemotherapy. The treatment decision relies on the size, location, growth, metastasis of the tumor and the age and health of the patient.

Like other cancers, treatment of lung cancer can also be curative (tumor surgery or radiation) or palliative (*if the treatment of cancer is not possible, then therapy given to reduce pain and discomfort is called palliative treatment*). More than one kind of treatment is usually given. When a treatment is given to increase the effect of the main treatment, then it is called **adjuvant therapy**. For example, chemotherapy or radiotherapy is given as adjuvant therapy to kill the remaining cancer cells after surgery. If treatment is given to reduce tumors before surgery, then it is called **neo adjuvant therapy**.

Surgery

Removal of tumor by surgery is the most appropriate treatment, if the cancer has not spread outside the lungs. This surgery is done in early stage (stage I or sometimes stage II) of non-small cell cancers. Generally, surgery is possible in only 10% -35% of non-small cell cancer patients. But the patient is not able to get complete relief if cancer has already spread at the time of diagnosis and after surgery, the cancer may recur any time. If surgery is performed in patients with slow growing solitary cancer, only 25%-40% of them may survive for five years. Many times the patient is stage wise suitable candidate for surgery cancer, but due to a serious condition of the patient (such as a major disease of the heart or lungs) surgery can be a risky task.

The possibility of surgery in small cell cancers is relatively limited, because it spreads rapidly and does not stay confined in one part of the lungs.

Surgery depends on the size and location of the tumor. This is a major surgery, the patient has to be admitted and after surgery, he has to stay in the hospital for a long time. In this surgery, the patient is given general anesthesia and chest has to be opened. After this, the surgeon removes a small portion of the lung i.e. **wedge resection** is done. Sometimes a lobe is removed **(lobectomy)** or complete lung is removed **(pneumonectomy)**. Sometimes lymph nodes located in the lung are also removed. After surgery, the patient suffers from difficulty in breathing, pain and weakness. Bleeding, infection and side-effects of anesthesia are the main hazards of surgery.

Radiotherapy

Radiotherapy is given in both small cell and non-small cell cancers. In this treatment powerful X-rays or other types of radiation is used to kill rapidly dividing cancer cells. Radiotherapy is given as **curative, palliative** or **adjuvant therapy** with other treatments (surgery or chemo). Most often, radiation therapy is delivered by the external beam technique, which aims a beam of x-rays directly at the tumor or by Brachytherapy.

In **Brachytherapy** small pallets filled with radioactive substances, is kept near the lump or in a nearby airway by a bronchoscope. Also, in the setting of an obstructive tumor within an airway, radiation is delivered to the site of obstruction through a plastic tube that is temporarily inserted into the airway. This may help to relieve severe symptoms but does not cure the cancer. In this, the radiation from the pellet travels a small distance, so the damage to the surrounding healthy tissues is very small. Brachytherapy is suitable in treating the symptoms of cancer due to the presence of tumors located in airways.

If the patient refuses for surgery or his cancer has already spread to lymph nodes and/or airways that surgery is not possible or patient is not fit for surgery because he has some serious heart or lung disease, then he is given radiotherapy. When the radiation is given as a main treatment, it only makes the lump smaller or limits its growth, so that the patient remains healthy for some time. 10% -15% of patients live a healthy life for a fairly long time.

Chemotherapy is also given with radiotherapy, so the life expectancy increases slightly. External beam radiotherapy is given in the O.P.D. department, but to provide internal radiotherapy, the patient has to be admitted for a day or two. If the patient has a serious lung disease along with cancer, then the radiotherapy can't be given because it can damage the lung. A special type of gamma knife is used to give radiotherapy to the solitary metastatic tumor in the brain. By stabilizing the head, radiation is given for several minutes or hours by focusing on several beams of the radiation. In this healthy tissues gets a relatively small amount of radiation.

Prior to external radiotherapy, simulation procedure is done to find out where the radiation should be concentrated, with the help of C.T. Scan, computer and correct measurements. It takes about 30 minutes to two hours. External radiation is given 4 or 5 days a week for several weeks.

Radiation therapy does not have serious side-effects like surgery, but there are some unpleasant effects such as fatigue and weakness. Lowering white blood cells (there is a risk of infection) or decrease of platelets (there is a risk of bleeding) are also the effects of radiation. Radiation also affects the digestive organs, and nausea, vomiting or diarrhea may occur. Skin may have itching and irritation.

Chemotherapy

Chemotherapy is given in both small cell and non-small cell cancers. However, nowadays many chemotherapeutic drugs are used, but platinum based drugs such as cisplatin or carboplatin have proved to be more effective in lung cancer. Chemotherapy is the only treatment left for almost all small cell cancers, because at the time of diagnosis it has often spread throughout the body. Half of the small cell cancer patients hardly live four months without chemotherapy. But after the chemo, his life may be prolonged. The single drug chemotherapy has not proved to be so effective in non-small cell cancers, but if the cancer has metastasized then the lifespan of many patients might prolong.

Chemotherapy refers to the use of cytotoxic (cell-killing) medications to kill cancer cells or make them less active, and is often used with lung cancer. Not all medications used now for lung cancer are considered chemotherapy, and targeted therapies and immunotherapy drugs work by a different mechanism. Chemotherapy may be used as after surgery to treat any remaining cells (adjunct chemotherapy), or for metastatic lung cancer to extend life. It also now used along with treatments such as immunotherapy to increase the effectiveness of these drugs.

How Chemotherapy Works

Chemotherapy medications work by killing rapidly dividing cells. Since cancer cells divide more frequently than most cells, they are particularly susceptible to these drugs. Some normal cells also divide continuously, such as hair follicles, the stomach lining, and the bone marrow that makes red and white blood cells. This accounts for many of the side effects experienced during chemotherapy, such as hair loss, nausea, and low blood cell counts. Different chemotherapy medications work at different stages of cell division. For this reason, often two or more medications are given at the same time to kill as many cancer cells as possible (combination chemotherapy). Understanding cancer cells, and the differences between cancer cells and normal cells, can help you understand a little easier how chemotherapy works.

Unlike surgery and radiation therapy, which are considered "local" treatments, chemotherapy is a "systemic treatment," meaning that it works to kill cancer cells anywhere in the body. This can be particularly helpful if cancer cells may have spread beyond the regions treated by surgery and radiation. Chemotherapy may be considered for several reasons:

- As an adjunct to surgery: In this case, chemotherapy is given to kill any cancer cells that may have spread beyond the cancer but are undetectable by scans. This is often referred to as adjuvant chemotherapy.
- To shrink a tumor before surgery: In some cases, chemotherapy is used before surgery to shrink a tumor and improve the chances that surgery will be effective. This method is often referred to as **neoadjuvant chemotherapy.**
- To prolong life in those with advanced lung cancer: Often chemotherapy can extend life when a cure is not possible. When chemotherapy has been effective in reducing the size of a tumor, a smaller dose of chemotherapy is sometimes used in the hope that it will delay the recurrent growth of a tumor. This is referred to as maintenance chemotherapy.
- To help with symptoms of cancer: When a tumor is causing symptoms such as pain or shortness of breath, sometimes chemotherapy can reduce the size of the tumor to decrease symptoms.
- To make immunotherapy drugs work better: Immunotherapy drugs work simplistically but stimulating the immune system to fight cancer. In order for these drugs to work, the immune cells need to be "familiar" with the cancer cells, or recognize antigens (protein markers) on the surface. Cancer cells have ways of "hiding" so that they are not recognized. Chemotherapy drugs can break down cancer cells, releasing pieces into the circulation. The immune cells that are stimulated by immunotherapy drugs can then better recognize their targets.

When chemotherapy is given for symptoms alone (to improve quality of life) and not with an intent to cure the disease or lengthen survival, it is referred to as palliative chemotherapy. If your doctor is offering chemotherapy in this way, make sure he discusses this carefully with you, as studies suggest many people are confused about the reason behind its use.

How Chemotherapy Is Given

Some chemotherapy medications are given as an oral pill, but most are given intravenously. If you will be having IV chemotherapy, you may be asked to make a choice between having an IV placed at each visit, or having a chemotherapy port placed. With a port, an intravenous line is threaded into the large blood vessels near the top of the chest, and a small metal or plastic device is placed under your skin. There are advantages and disadvantages to each method, yet a port (or sometimes a PICC line) can reduce the number of needle pricks necessary during treatment.

The initial treatment for lung cancer usually involves the use of 2 or more drugs (combination chemotherapy). These drugs are often given in cycles of 3 to 4 weeks at least 4 to 6 times. Using a combination of drugs which work at different phases of cell division increases the chance of treating as many cancer cells as possible. Since different cells are all in different places in the process of cell division, repeated sessions also increase the chance of treating as many cancer cells as possible.

Medications

Chemotherapy has not proved to be very effective in non-small cell lung cancer. Often, one of the following medicines is given with cisplatin or Carboplatin (paraplatin).

- **Vinorelbine**
- **Gemcitabine**
- **Paclitaxel (Taxol)**
- **Docetaxel (Taxotere)**

- **Doxorubicin**
- **Etoposide**
- **Pametrexade**
- **Ifosfamide**
- **Mitomycin**
- **Topotecan**

Non-Cytotoxic Cancer Medications

Not all medications used for lung cancer are considered chemotherapy. Medications such as Tarceva (erlotinib) and Xalkori (crizotinib) are targeted therapy drugs, medications designed to specifically treat cancer cells. A relatively new category of medications, called immunotherapy drugs, is now also being used for lung cancer. These drugs work simplistically by helping our immune systems fight cancer.

Regimens of chemotherapy

The prevailing regimens of chemotherapy in small cell lung cancers are as follows.
- **PE regimen**
  Cisplatin 25 mg / m^2 IV days 1-3
  Etoposide 100 mg / m^2 IV days 1-3
- **PEC regimen**
  Paclitaxel 200 mg / m2 IV day 1
  Etoposide 50 mg / d PO alternating with
      100 mg / d PO from days 1-10
  Carboplatin AUC 6 IV day 1
- **CAV regimen**
  Cyclophosphamide 1000 mg / m2 IV day 1
  Doxorubicin 50 mg / m2 IV day 1
  Vincristine 2 mg IV
- **CAVE**
  Cyclophosphamide 1000 mg / m2 IV day 1
  Doxorubicin 50 mg / m2 IV day 1
  Vincristine 2mg IV
  Itoposide 100 mg / m2 IV day 1

- **Single drug regimen**
  Topotecan 1.5 mg / m2 IV day 1-5
  Etoposide 50 mg PO bid days 1-14

The following chemotherapy is given in recurrent cancer.
- **ACE** (doxorubicin, cyclophosphamide and etoposide) or
- **CAV** (Cyclophosphamide, Doxorubicin and Vincristine)

Topotecan if patient suffers from heart disease and it is not possible to doxorubicin, as it damages the heart.

AUC = area under the concentration curve; bid = twice daily; IV = administered intravenously; PO = administered orally

Why Can't Chemotherapy Cure Lung Cancer?

If you are familiar with chemotherapy agents used for leukemia, which can often cure the disease, you may wonder why chemotherapy does not usually cure lung cancer. This can be even more confusing when you see that chemotherapy is often effective early on for lung cancer in that it can significantly shrink a tumor. This question is important to address as many people feel chemotherapy has the strong potential to cure their cancer.

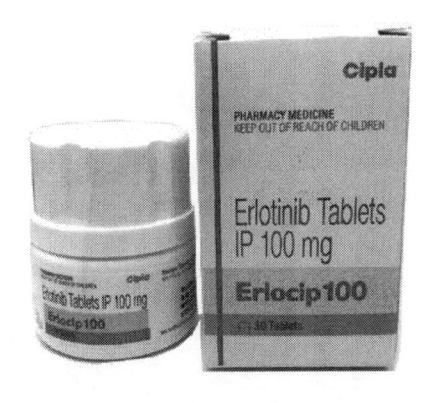

The reason why chemotherapy does not usually cure lung cancer is that tumors become resistant to the drugs over time. Cancer cells are "smart" in a way. They do not stay the same, but constantly change and develop methods for escaping the treatments we send their way. Resistance is one reason why -

when someone has a tumor which has begun to grow again on chemotherapy; different drugs are often used the next time around.

Side Effects of Chemotherapy

Side effects of chemotherapy vary depending on the medications you are given, and other factors such as your age, sex, and general medical condition. Thankfully, management of these side effects has made tremendous strides over the past few decades. Everyone responds to chemotherapy differently. You may have few side effects or you may instead find the symptoms quite troubling. These side effects can improve over time or worsen over time. Sometimes a medication may need to be changed, but often there are medications and treatments that can control your symptoms and make you more comfortable. Make sure to share any symptoms you are experiencing with your health care team.

Before beginning treatment, it's also important to understand the potential long term side effects of chemotherapy. As noted, many of these side effects are related to the "normal" effect of chemotherapy on rapidly dividing cells. Cells in our bodies which divide most rapidly include those in our bone marrow (leading to low blood counts) our hair follicles, and our digestive tracts. The most common side effect of chemotherapy includes:

- **Nausea and Vomiting:** Nausea and vomiting are quite common on chemotherapy, but the management of these side effects has improved dramatically in recent years. It is now possible for many people to go through chemotherapy treatment with minimal or no nausea or vomiting. Often medications are given not only to treat nausea but given along with chemotherapy to prevent nausea.
- **Mouth Sores:** Roughly half of people develop mouth sores on chemotherapy for lung cancer. These mouth

sores are most often more of a nuisance, but secondary infections (thrush) may sometimes develop.
- **Taste Changes:** An abnormal sense of taste, often referred to as "metal mouth" is common with lung cancer chemotherapy drugs. There are several things you can do that may help you better tolerate this symptom.
- **Loss of Appetite:** Loss of appetite is extremely important to address, as getting adequate nutrition during chemotherapy can help your body heal. An inadequate intake of nutrients can also place you at risk of cancer cachexia - a syndrome of weight loss and muscle wasting that is directly responsible for nearly 20 percent of cancer deaths.
- **Fatigue:** Fatigue is the most common side effect of chemotherapy, affecting nearly everyone at some point. Simply recognizing that fatigue is common, and learning to prioritize activities and accept help is often the best solution for coping with this annoying side effect.
- **Anemia** (low red blood cell count): A low red blood cell count can lead to fatigue. Sometimes treatment is needed, but as with fatigue, often learning to ask for help and get more rest is all that is needed.
- **Neutropenia** (low white blood cell count): A low white blood cell count (neutrophils are a type of white blood cell which fights infection) is often the most serious side effect of chemotherapy. Having a low white blood cell count can predispose you to infections. Make sure to talk to your doctor about this before you begin chemotherapy. He may recommend that you avoid situations in which you could be predisposed to infections - such as avoiding crowds and minimizing contact with people who are sick. Sometimes medications are used which stimulate the production of white blood cells after chemotherapy. If your white blood cell count is too low, your

chemotherapy session may need to be delayed until it has returned to acceptable values.
- **Thrombocytopenia** (low platelet count): A low platelet count may result in easy bruising or bleeding. This is not often a serious concern with chemotherapy for lung cancer, but your doctor will monitor your platelet count carefully throughout your treatment.
- **Hair Loss:** Many of the chemotherapy drugs used for lung cancer can result in hair loss. Preparing ahead by purchasing a wig or other forms of head covers is often recommended. Doxorubicin (often called Red Devil) is notorious drug for causing hair loss.
- **Skin Changes**
- **Fingernail changes**
- **Depression**
- **Chemobrain** (cognitive changes after chemotherapy): Chemobrain, or cognitive changes after chemotherapy has recently been recognized as a fairly common side effect of chemotherapy. Common symptoms include difficulty multitasking or mild forgetfulness - such as forgetting where you placed the car keys. Some people find that "brain exercises" such as doing crossword puzzles and other logic games is helpful if this becomes bothersome.
- **Peripheral Neuropathy:** Peripheral neuropathy is quite common for people going through chemotherapy for lung cancer. Symptoms can include pain and tingling in what is called a "*stocking and gloves*" distribution. Research is ongoing looking for methods to not only relieve the symptoms of this side effect but to prevent it from occurring in the first place.

Support and Coping During Chemotherapy

Certainly, there are side effects with chemotherapy, but the management of these has improved significantly in recent years.

Chemotherapy is one of those times when the adage "it takes a village" is as true as ever. Reach out to family and friends and allow people to help you. Many people find it helpful to join a cancer support group or support community and have the opportunity to talk to others who are experiencing similar challenges in their lives. Since most people have several chemotherapy sessions, and these sessions take some time, this can be a chance to reconnect with family and friends. Check out this list of what to pack for chemotherapy for ideas on how to make your chemotherapy sessions go as smoothly as possible.

Radiation of the Brain

Small cell cancers often spread in the brain. Therefore, many times a small cell cancer patient is given protective radiotherapy to kill cancer cells (called micrometastasis), even if there is no visible metastasis in the brain and C.T. or M.R.I. scan doesn't show any signs of metastasis. There are some short-term side effects such as short-term memory loss, fatigue, vomiting, etc. to give the brain radiation.

Treatment of Recurrent Cancer

Lung cancer is more likely to recur in the first five years following diagnosis. This is why it's important to have regular check-ups.

If the cancer returns, your doctor will discuss the treatment options with you. These will depend on the type of lung cancer and where the cancer has recurred, as well as the stage and grade of the cancer. You may be offered radiation therapy, chemotherapy or the option to join a clinical trial. If you have recurrent non-small cell lung cancer, you may also be offered targeted therapy.

Photodynamic Treatment (PDT)

This is a new treatment for lungs and many other cancers, and can be given in all types and all stages. In this, a photosensitizing substance is injected in the vein a few hours before the procedure. The agent is absorbed by cells all over the body but stays in cancer cells longer than it does in normal cells. Approximately 24 to 72 hours after injection, when most of the agent has left normal cells but remains in cancer cells, the tumor is exposed to light. The photo sensitizer in the tumor absorbs the light and produces an active form of oxygen that destroys nearby cancer cells.

In addition to directly killing cancer cells, PDT appears to shrink or destroy tumors in two other ways. The photosensitizer can damage blood vessels in the tumor, thereby preventing the cancer from receiving necessary nutrients. PDT also may activate the immune system to attack the tumor cells.

The light used for PDT can come from a laser or other sources. Laser light can be directed through fiber optic cable (thin fibers that transmit light) to deliver light to areas inside the body. For example, a fiber optic cable can be inserted through an endoscope (a thin, lighted tube used to look at tissues inside the body) into the lungs to treat cancer in these organs. Other light sources include light-emitting diodes (LEDs), which may be used for surface tumors, such as skin cancer.

PDT is less invasive and usually performed as an outpatient procedure. PDT may also be repeated and may be used with other therapies, such as surgery, radiation therapy, or chemotherapy.

Recently, mono-l-aspartyl chlorine e6 (NPe6, Laserphyrin), a second-generation photosensitizer with lower photosensitivity than Photofrin (porfimer sodium), was approved by the Japanese government and a phase II clinical study using NPe6 with a new diode laser demonstrated an excellent antitumor effect and low skin photosensitivity.

Radio Frequency Ablation (RFA)

Radio Frequency Ablation Treatment has emerged as a substitute for surgery for early lung cancers that are near the outer edge of the lungs. RFA uses high-energy radio waves to heat the tumor. A thin, needle-like probe is put through the skin and moved in until the tip is in the tumor. Placement of the probe is guided by CT scan. Once the tip is in place, an electric current is passed through the probe, which heats the tumor and destroys the cancer cells and block the veins that supply the blood to the cancer. This is usually painless treatment and FDA Certified for many cancers including lung cancer. RFA is usually done as an outpatient procedure, using local anesthesia. You may be given medicine to help you relax as well. The treatment is as effective as surgery and the risk is very low.

You might have some pain where the needle was inserted for a few days after the procedure. Major complications are uncommon, but they can include the partial collapse of a lung (which often goes away on its own) or bleeding into the lung.

Clinical trials

There is no successful treatment for lung cancer in conventional oncology. Therefore, the patient can also take new clinical trials. Because these treatments are in an experimental stage and physicians do not have enough information about how safe these treatments are and how effective they are. *Therefore, patient can take this treatment at his own risk.*

Targeted Therapy

Targeted therapy works by targeting the cancer's specific genes, proteins, or the tissue environment that contributes to cancer growth and survival. These genes and proteins are found in cancer cells or in cells related to cancer growth, like blood vessel cells.

Doctors often use targeted therapy with chemotherapy and other treatments. The U.S. Food and Drug Administration (FDA) have approved targeted therapies for many types of cancer. Scientists are also testing drugs for new cancer targets.

Prior to taking targeted therapy, the cancer tissue samples are examined and it is found out which type of mutation is present in the tumor. Targeted drug is selected based on this testing. About

14 US institutes are doing this test for free for cancer patients. Although many mutations have been marked so far, but the targeted drugs have not been developed so far. Nowadays, three types of mutations are examined EGFR, ALK and KRAS.

There is an EGFR mutation in about 20% to 30% of adenocarcinoma sub-type of non-small cell cancers. In this, Tarceva and Iressa target medicines are given. These are tyrosine kinase Inhibitors. Targeted therapy is particularly targeted to cancer cells, resulting in relatively less damage to normal cells. Arlotinib and Jeffitinib target upon epidermal growth factor receptor (EGFR) protein. This protein helps in increasing the division of cells. This protein is present in large quantities on the surface of many cancer cells such as non-small cell cancer cells. These are given in the form of tablets. These increases the life expectancy of cancer patients with EGFR mutations, but after some time the patient gets resistance from this drug.

Tarceva works by not allowing EGFR to tell cancer cells to grow. While potentially effective in many kinds of patients, it has been shown to be more likely to work for those who have never smoked or in younger women. Given as a daily pill, the most common side effects are a skin rash similar to acne, and diarrhea. Though the skin rash can be a cosmetic nuisance, those who develop a rash with erlotinib are more likely to be responding to therapy. EGFR inhibitors used in NSCLC with EGFR gene mutations are as follows:

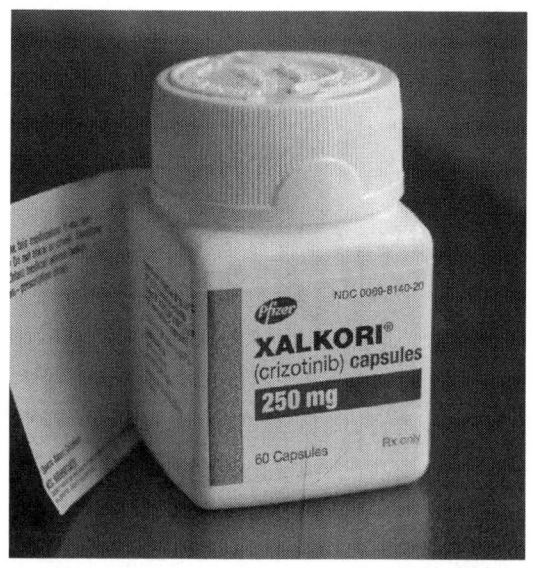

- **Erlotinib (Tarceva)**
- **Afatinib (Gilotrif)**
- **Gefitinib (Iressa)**
- **Osimertinib (Tagrisso)**
- **Dacomitinib (Vizimpro)**

These drugs can be used alone (without chemo) as the first treatment for advanced NSCLCs that have certain mutations in the EGFR gene. These are more common in women and people who haven't smoked. Erlotinib can also be used for advanced NSCLC without these mutations if chemo isn't working. All of these medicines are taken as pills.

About 2% to 7% of non-small cell cancers have an ALC (anaplastic lymphoma kinase) mutation. These patients are often young and do not smoke (except 1-2%). For this, a new target drug Crizotinib (crizotinib) has been approved. It neutralizes the ALK and prevents growth of cancer cells. It reduces the tumor and may keeps it stable for about 6 months. This drug, manufactured by the Pfizer company, is available in the name of Xalcori. Drugs that target the abnormal ALK protein include:

- **Crizotinib (Xalkori)**
- **Ceritinib (Zykadia)**
- **Alectinib (Alecensa)**
- **Brigatinib (Alunbrig)**
- **Lorlatinib (Lorbrena)**

These drugs can often shrink tumors in people whose lung cancers have the ALK gene change. Although they can help after chemo has stopped working, they are often used instead of chemo in people whose cancers have the ALK gene rearrangement.

At least some of these drugs also seem to be useful in treating people whose cancers have changes in the ROS1 gene.

These drugs are taken as pills and are very costly.

Side effects

Common side effects of ALK inhibitors include:

- Nausea and vomiting
- Diarrhea
- Constipation
- Fatigue
- Changes in vision

Other side effects are also possible with some of these drugs. Some side effects can be severe, such as low white blood cell counts, inflammation (swelling) in the lungs or other parts of the body, liver damage, nerve damage (peripheral neuropathy), and heart rhythm problems.

Setuximab is an antibody that is linked to the epidermal growth factor receptor. If this EGFR is pervasive on the surface of non-small cell cancers, then Satuximab may be beneficial.

Drugs that target tumor blood vessel growth (angiogenesis)

For tumors to grow, they need to form new blood vessels to keep them nourished. This process is called angiogenesis. Some targeted drugs, called angiogenesis inhibitors, block this new blood vessel growth:

Bevacizumab (Avastin) is used to treat advanced NSCLC. It is a monoclonal antibody (a man-made version of a specific immune system protein) that targets vascular endothelial growth factor (VEGF), a protein that helps new blood vessels to form. This drug is often used with chemo for a time. Then if the cancer responds, the chemo may be stopped and the bevacizumab given by itself until the cancer starts growing again. There is a risk of bleeding from this drug, so patients should not be given if he coughs out blood, who are taking anticoagulation medication or their cancer has spread in the brain. It should not be given in squamous cell carcinoma as it has a risk of bleeding.

Ramucirumab (Cyramza) can also be used to treat advanced NSCLC. VEGF has to bind to cell proteins called receptors to act. This drug is a monoclonal antibody that targets a VEGF receptor. This helps stop the formation of new blood vessels. This drug is most often given after another treatment stops working. It is often combined with chemo.

Side effects

Common side effects of these drugs include:
- High blood pressure
- Tiredness (fatigue)
- Bleeding
- Low white blood cell counts (with increased risk of infections)
- Headaches
- Mouth sores
- Loss of appetite
- Diarrhea

Rare but possibly serious side effects can include blood clots, severe bleeding, perforations in the intestine, heart problems, and slow wound healing. If a perforation forms in the intestine it can lead to severe infection and may require surgery to correct.

Because of the risks of bleeding, these drugs typically aren't used in people who are coughing up blood or who are taking drugs called blood thinners. The risk of serious bleeding in the lungs is higher in patients with the squamous cell type of NSCLC, which is why most current guidelines do not recommend using bevacizumab in people with this type of lung cancer.

Drugs that target cells with BRAF gene changes

In some NSCLCs, the cells have changes in the BRAF gene. Cells with these changes make an altered BRAF protein that helps them grow. Some drugs target this and related proteins:

Dabrafenib (Tafinlar) is a type of drug known as a BRAF inhibitor, which attacks the BRAF protein directly.

Trametinib (Mekinist) is known as a MEK inhibitor, because it attacks the related MEK proteins.

These drugs can be used together to treat metastatic NSCLC if it has a certain type of BRAF gene change. These drugs are taken as pills or capsules each day.

Side effects

Common side effects can include skin thickening, rash, itching, and sensitivity to the sun, headache, fever, joint pain, fatigue, hair loss, nausea, and diarrhea.

Less common but serious side effects can include bleeding, heart rhythm problems, liver or kidney problems, lung problems, severe allergic reactions, severe skin or eye problems, and increased blood sugar levels.

Some people treated with these drugs develop skin cancers, especially squamous cell skin cancers. Your doctor will want to check your skin often during treatment and for several months afterward. You should also let your doctor know right away if you notice any new growths or abnormal areas on your skin.

Lung Cancer Prognosis

There are many different types of lung cancer, but the two main types are small cell lung cancer (SCLC) and non-small cell lung cancer (NSCLC). About 15% of lung cancers are SCLC, while 85% are NSCLC.

SCLC grows quickly and has often already reached an advanced stage when it is diagnosed. NSCLC, on the other hand, is more slow growing and may be diagnosed at a stage when it can be surgically removed. The outlook after treatment for patients with these forms of lung cancer is described below.

Non-small cell lung cancer

There are four main stages to lung cancer and in 2007, a study called the Lung Cancer Staging Project gathered data for 81,000 lung cancer patients and gave survival statistics for people with different stages of NSCLC. For each stage, the cancer is further divided into stages A and B.

Stage 1

This first stage of the disease is associated with the best treatment outcome because it is often possible to surgically remove stage 1 tumors. Between 59% and 73% of people with stage 1A will survive for at least 5 years after diagnosis, while for those with stage 1B, the figure is between 43% and 58%.

Stage 2

For stage 2A, it is projected that between 36% and 46% will survive for at least five years or more after diagnosis if they receive treatment, while for stage 2 B, this figure is between 25% and 36%.

Stage 3

The survival statistics start to fall with more advanced stages of lung cancer. For stage 3A, the five year survival rate after diagnosis is between 19% and 24%, while for those with stage 3B, the figure is 7% to 9%.

Stage 4

This the most advanced stage of lung cancer, when the cancer has spread beyond the lung to other parts of the body. The survival statistics for stage 4 lung cancer are very low. For individuals with stage 4 disease, only between 2 and 13% will survive for at least five years after diagnosis.

Small cell lung cancer

Small cell lung cancer is sometimes divided into two groups: limited disease, which describes cancer that has not yet spread beyond the lung and extensive disease, where the cancer has spread beyond the lung.

Around 30% of people diagnosed with small cell lung cancer have limited disease when the cancer is diagnosed and, with treatment, around one quarter of those will survive for at least 2 years. Two thirds of individuals with small cell lung cancer already have extensive disease when their condition is diagnosed. The chances of survival are low and even with treatment, less than 5% survive for at least 5 years after diagnosis.

Below, are survival statistics generated by the Lung Cancer Staging Project based on stage for 8,000 patients with small cell lung cancer.

Stage 1

Of patients diagnosed with stage 1A, 40% will survive for at least 5 years after diagnosis, while for those with stage 1B, the figure is 20%.

Stage 2

Of patients diagnosed with stage 2A, around 40% will survive for at least 5 years after diagnosis, while for those diagnosed with stage 2B, the figure is 20%.

Stage 3

Again, at this stage, the survival statistics are less optimistic. For stage 3A, the percentage of patients who will survive for at least five years after diagnosis is 15%, while for stage 3B, the figure is 10%.

Stage 4

Here, the cancer has already spread beyond the lung to other parts of the body. Since lung cancer tends to only get diagnosed in the late stages, unfortunately, the cancer has often already spread at the time of diagnosis. Only around 1% of people with stage 4 disease will survive for at least 5 years after diagnosis.

Can Lung Cancer Be Prevented?

Not all lung cancers can be prevented. But there are things you can do that might lower your risk, such as changing the risk factors that you can control.

Stay away from tobacco

The best way to reduce your risk of lung cancer is not to smoke and to avoid breathing in other people's smoke.

If you stop smoking before a cancer develops, your damaged lung tissue gradually starts to repair itself. No matter what your age or how long you've smoked, quitting may lower your risk of lung cancer and help you live longer.

Limiting your exposure to second hand smoke might also help lower your risk of lung cancer, as well as some other cancers.

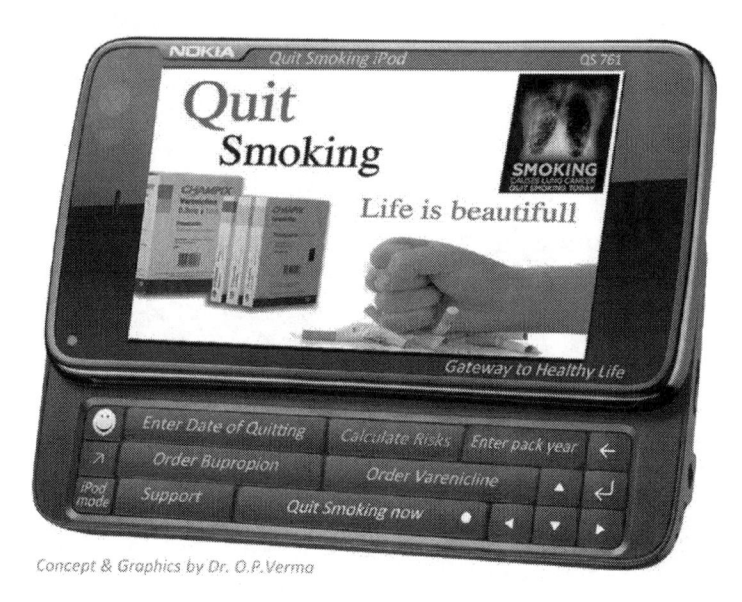

Concept & Graphics by Dr. O.P.Verma

Consume Flax Oil and healthy diet

Consume only Flax oil as oil. Avoid frozen and preserved meat. Fresh meat is OK. No frozen food and no bakery products. Avoid all Trans fats. Eat organic diet. Oleolox should be used as butter. Prepare fruit juices yourself. Cheese and potatoes are OK. Also the electromagnetic environment (e.g. microwave and mobile phones etc.) in which we live is very important. I reject synthetic textiles and foam mattresses because they steal lot of electrons from you. The environment and living conditions must be as biological (organic & natural) as possible.

Avoid radon

Radon is an important cause of lung cancer. You can reduce your exposure to radon by having your home tested and treated, if needed.

Avoid or limit exposure to cancer-causing chemicals

Avoiding exposure to known cancer-causing chemicals, in the workplace and elsewhere, may also be helpful. When people work where these exposures are common, they should be kept to a minimum.

Alternative cancer treatments

We are fighting with cancer since the dawn of history. Every year we discover new diagnostic modalities, better radiotherapy techniques and lots of new chemotherapy drugs. But we have completely failed to defeat this disease called cancer. Think again, are we really going on the right path? Does conventional Medicine really targets upon the prime cause of cancer?

It's not that more effective alternative treatments for cancer don't exist – they most certainly do. It's just that the allopathic system isn't at all interested in divulging real cures. This is because their expensive therapies generate billions of dollars for the cancer industry.

Chemotherapy Doesn't Cure Cancer – It Causes It!

Chemotherapy does, in fact, kill cancer cells. But it also kills healthy cells, along with a patient's immune system and, really, anything else that crosses its path. At worst, such treatments kill patients more quickly than if they had chosen not to undergo them at all.

There's no money to be made in prescribing prevention advice like eating fewer chemicals and exercising more. The "bread and butter" of the cancer industry is unleashing the next, latest-and-greatest cancer drug. Not telling you how to avoid cancer in the first place.

Many people with cancer are interested in trying any treatment that may cure them safely, including complementary and alternative cancer treatments. There is growing evidence that these alternative cancer treatments give wonderful results. Here are some alternative cancer treatments that are very safe and effective.

- **Budwig Protocol -** *The best Alternative Treatment effective in all cancersand all stages with documented 90% success*

- Laetrile (Vitamin B-17) Therapy
- Gerson Therapy
- Dr. Simoncini Baking Soda Cancer Treatment
- High-dose vitamin C
- Frankincense Essential Oil Therapy
- Immunotherapy
- Hyperthermia
- Oxygen Therapy and Hyperbaric Chambers

Laetrile (Vitamin B-17) Therapy

Introduction

During 1950, after many years of research, a dedicated biochemist Dr. Ernest T. Krebs Jr., isolated a new vitamin from bitter apricot kernel that he called 'B-17' or 'Laetrile'. He conducted further lab animal and culture experiments to conclude that laetrile would be effective in the treatment of cancer. As the years rolled by, thousands became convinced that Krebs had finally found the treatment for all cancers. He proposed that cancer was caused by a deficiency of Vitamin B 17 (Laetrile, Amygdaline).

To prove that it was not toxic to humans he injected it into his own arm. As he predicted, there were no harmful or distressing side effects. The Laetrile had no harmful effect on normal cells but was deadly to cancer cells. Dr. Ernst Krebs stated that we need at least a minimum of 100 mg of B-17 or around 7 bitter apricot seeds to almost guarantee a cancer free life.

Nitriloside is a beta-cyanophoric glycosides, a large group of water-soluble, sugar-containing compounds found in a number of plants. Amygdalin is one of the most common nitrilosides. Laetrile is a partly man-made molecule and shares only part of the Amygdalin structure. Both Laetrile and Amygdalin have been promoted as "Vitamin B-17".

Laetrile stands for laevo-rotatory mandelonitrile beta-diglucoside. The "laevo" part references a purified form of B-17 that turns polarized light in a left-turning direction. Dr. Krebs, Jr. believed that only the left-rotating Laevo form was effective against cancer. So it's important to check the purity of your Laetrile.

How B-17 works (A tale of two enzymes)

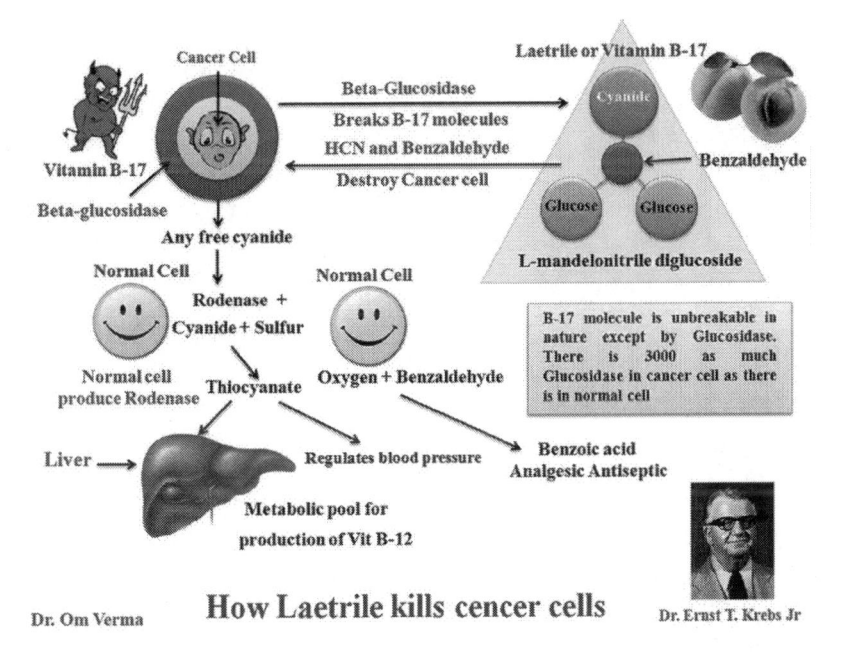

Cancer Cell — Beta-Glucosidase Breaks B-17 molecules HCN and Benzaldehyde Destroy Cancer cell

Laetrile or Vitamin B-17 — Cyanide, Benzaldehyde, Glucose, Glucose, L-mandelonitrile diglucoside

Vitamin B-17, Beta-glucosidase

Any free cyanide

Normal Cell — Rodenase + Cyanide + Sulfur

Normal cell produce Rodenase — Thiocyanate

Normal Cell — Oxygen + Benzaldehyde

B-17 molecule is unbreakable in nature except by Glucosidase. There is 3000 as much Glucosidase in cancer cell as there is in normal cell

Liver → Regulates blood pressure

Metabolic pool for production of Vit B-12

Benzoic acid Analgesic Antiseptic

Dr. Om Verma — **How Laetrile kills cencer cells** — Dr. Ernst T. Krebs Jr

Laetrile, commonly known as Vitamin B-17 or Amygdalin, contains two units of Sugar, one of Benzaldehyde and one of Cyanide, all tightly locked within it. Everyone knows that cyanide can be highly toxic and even fatal if taken in sufficient quantity. However, as it is in locked state is completely inert and absolutely has no effect on living tissue. There is only one substance that can unlock this molecule and release the cyanide. That substance is an enzyme called beta-glucocidase, which we shall call the unlocking enzyme. When B-17 comes in contact with this enzyme, not only the cyanide is released but also Benzaldehyde which is highly toxic by itself. In fact, these two working together are at least 100 times more poisonous to cancer cell than either of them separately. The unlocking enzyme is not found to any dangerous degree anywhere in the body except at the cancer cell where it is present in great quantity. The result is that Vit B-17 is unlocked at the cancer cells becomes poisonous to the cancer cells and only to the cancer cells.

There is another important enzyme called Rodanese, which we shall identify as protecting enzyme. The reason is that it has the ability to neutralize cyanide by converting it instantly into the byproducts (thiocyanate) that actually are beneficial and essential for health. This enzyme is found in great quantities in every part of the body except the cancer cells which consequently is not protected. Here then is a biochemical process that destroys cancer cells while at the same time nourishing and sustaining non-cancerous cells. It is intricate and perfect mechanism of nature that simply couldn't be accidental.

Laetrile - Metabolic Therapy

Metabolic therapy is a non-toxic cancer treatment based on the use of Vitamin B- 17, proteolytic pancreatic enzymes, immuno-stimulants, and vitamin and mineral supplements.

There are three parts to this program:
1. Laetrile
2. Vitamins and enzymes
3. Diet

Phase I Metabolic - Program for the first 21 days

Laetrile

Amygdalin (Laetrile) is available in 500 mg. tablets and in vials (10 cc 3 Gm) for intravenous use. Both forms are used. Two vials of Laetrile are given IV three times weekly for three weeks with at least one day between injections (Mon., Wed., Fri.). Dose of Amygdalin Tablets 500 mg is 2 tab three times a day with meals on the days on which the patients do not receive the intravenous Laetrile. Thiocyanate levels in the blood can be measured during treatment. In general, the patients who do best are those in whom the thiocyanate level is between 1.2 and 2.5 Mg/DL (Philip E.Binzel).

Vitamins and Enzymes

Preven-Ca Caps - Preven-Ca is a comprehensive blend of potent herb and fruit extracts, designed to provide a broad Spectrum of Flavonoids with scientifically demonstrated Antioxidant activity and effectiveness. One capsule with each meal.

Vitamin B15 - One capsule three times a daily at the end of each meal.

Megazyme Forte (Proteolytic Enzymes) Three tablets two hours after each meal (9 daily).

Ester Vitamin C 1000 mg capsule - One capsule with each meal.

Shark Cartilage It has been said that Sharks are the healthiest creature on earth. Sharks are immune to practically every disease known to man. One capsules three times a daily with each meal.

Natural Vitamin E 400 iu - One gel with lunch and one with dinner.

AHCC (Active Hexose Correlated Compound) - Two capsules with each meal.

Multi Vitamin & Mineral Liquid - 1 oz (two tablespoons) once daily with a meal.

Vitamin A & E Emulsion - 5 drops in juice or water three times per day.

Barley Grass Juice - One teaspoon in juice three times per day.

Bitter apricot seeds - No more than 12 every 2 hours 6 times a day.

Dimethyl sulfoxide (DMSO) - DMSO is a by-product of the wood and paper industry. It is known for its ability to permeate living tissue and stimulate cellular processes.

Or Phase 1 Oral

Injectable Amygdalin is replaced with 500mg Amygdalin tablets. Binzel recommends 2 of these tablets with each meal for a total of 6 per day. Otherwise the ORAL Phase 1 includes the same materials as above.

Phase 2 Metabolic - Program for the next 3 months

It comprises the same materials as Phase 1 except that the dosages for the vitamin B-17 as well as the A&E Emulsion Drops change to the following:

Vitamin B-17 500 mg tablets: 1 tablet with each meal and one at bedtime.

Vitamin A & E emulsion drops: 10 drops in juice or water two times per day (suspend for 2 months after 3 months of use).

Diet

Consume those fruits (i.e. seeds), grains and nuts that are rich in laetrile. Consume salads with healthy dressings. For protein patient should consume whole grains including corn, beans, buckwheat, nuts, dried fruits. Real butter in small amounts is permitted. The patients are not permitted anything which contains white flour or white sugar. Take away all meat, all poultry, all fish, all eggs and milk from patients. Margarine is detrimental to good nutrition. No coffee is permitted.

Zinc acts as transport vehicle for laetrile in the body. If patient does not have sufficient zinc, laetrile will not get into the tissues of the body. That's why you should give a spoonful of pumpkin seeds along with bitter apricot kernels. The body will not rebuild any tissue without sufficient quantities of Vitamin C etc.

The Gerson Therapy

The Gerson Therapy is a natural treatment that activates the body's extraordinary ability to heal itself through an organic, plant-based diet, raw juices, coffee enemas and natural supplements.

With its whole-body approach to healing, the Gerson Therapy naturally reactivates your body's magnificent ability to heal itself – with no damaging side effects. This a powerful, natural treatment boosts the body's own immune system to heal cancer, arthritis, heart disease, allergies, and many other degenerative diseases. Dr. Max Gerson developed the Gerson Therapy in the 1930s, initially as a treatment for his own debilitating migraines, and eventually as a treatment for degenerative diseases such as skin tuberculosis, diabetes and, most famously, cancer.

An abundance of nutrients from copious amounts of fresh, organic juices are consumed every day, providing your body with a super-dose of enzymes, minerals and nutrients. These substances then break down diseased tissue in the body, while coffee enemas aid in eliminating toxins from the liver.

Throughout our lives our bodies are being filled with a variety of carcinogens and toxic pollutants. These toxins reach us through the air we breathe, the food we eat, the medicines we take and the water we drink. The Gerson Therapy's intensive detoxification regimen eliminates these toxins from the body, so that true healing can begin.

How the Gerson Therapy Works

The Gerson Therapy regenerates the body to health, supporting each important metabolic requirement by flooding the body with nutrients from about 15- 20 pounds of organically-grown fruits and vegetables daily. Most is used to make fresh raw juice, up to one glass every hour, up to 13 times per day. Raw and cooked solid foods are generously consumed. Oxygenation is usually more than doubled, as oxygen deficiency in the blood contributes to many degenerative diseases. The metabolism is also stimulated through the addition of thyroid, potassium and other supplements, and by avoiding heavy animal fats, excess protein, sodium and other toxins.

Degenerative diseases render the body increasingly unable to excrete waste materials adequately, commonly resulting in liver and kidney failure. The Gerson Therapy uses intensive detoxification to eliminate wastes, regenerate the liver, reactivate the immune system and restore the body's essential defenses – enzyme, mineral and hormone systems. With generous, high-quality nutrition, increased oxygen availability, detoxification, and improved metabolism, the cells – and the body – can regenerate, become healthy and prevent future illness.

Juicing

Fresh-pressed juice from raw foods provides the easiest and most effective way of providing high-quality nutrition. By juicing, patients can take in the nutrients and enzymes from nearly 15 pounds of produce every day, in a manner that is easy to digest and absorb.

Every day, a typical patient on the Gerson Therapy for cancer consumes up to thirteen glasses of fresh, raw carrot-apple and green leaf juices. These juices are prepared hourly from fresh, raw, organic fruits and vegetables, using a two-step juicer or a masticating juicer used with a separate hydraulic press.

The Gerson Therapy Diet

The Gerson Therapy diet is plant-based and entirely organic. The diet is naturally high in vitamins, minerals, enzymes, micro-nutrients, and extremely low in sodium, fats, and proteins. The following is a typical daily diet for a Gerson patient on the full therapy regimen:

- Thirteen glasses of fresh, raw carrot-apple and green-leaf juices prepared hourly from fresh, organic fruits and vegetables.
- Three full plant-based meals, freshly prepared from organically grown fruits, vegetables and whole grains. A typical meal will include salad, cooked vegetables, baked potatoes, Hippocrates soup and juice.
- Fresh fruit and vegetables available at all hours for snacking, in addition to the regular diet.

Supplements

All medications used in connection with the Gerson Therapy are classed as biologicals, materials of organic origin that are supplied in therapeutic amounts. The supplements used on the Gerson Therapy include:

- Potassium compound
- Lugol's solution
- Vitamin B-12
- Thyroid hormone
- Pancreatic Enzymes

Detoxification

Coffee enemas are the primary method of detoxification of the tissues and blood on the Gerson Therapy. Coffee enemas accomplish this essential task, assisting the liver in eliminating toxic residues from the body for good. Cancer patients on the Gerson Therapy may take up to 5 coffee enemas per day. The Gerson Therapy also utilizes castor oil to stimulate bile flow and enhance the liver's ability to filter blood.

Simoncini's Baking Soda Cancer Treatment

Dr. Tullio Simoncini is a medical doctor in Italy who has done more than anyone to explore the uses of the baking soda cancer treatment as an alternative cancer treatment. It is known that cancer creates and favors an acid environment and because of this, Dr. Simoncini and others have used sodium bicarbonate as an alkaline therapeutic agent.

The way that acidity seems to protect cancer is not fully understood. It seems that cytotoxic T-cells, which may attack cancer cells under normal conditions, are inactivated in an acid extracellular fluid. Also, the type of acidity that cancer produces, i.e., lactic acid, stimulates vascular endothelial growth factor and angiogenesis. This is like a highway project, which enables a tumor to build the blood vessels that it needs to bring the nutrients for it to survive. So the tumor creates an environment in which it can then exist comfortably.

Baking Soda's Alkalinity Fights Cancer's Acidity

At a pH of about 10, sodium bicarbonate is an antidote to this acidity. It can be used clinically in sterile, intravenous form. This is a liquid, sterile bicarbonate of soda. The baking soda cancer treatment is well-tolerated, even with frequent repeated dosing. Dr. Simonchini also injects soda bicarb solution directly into the tumors at his center.

Cancer a Fungus problem?

Dr. Simonchini says that cancer is caused by fungus However, it is useful to know that not only does sodium bicarbonate disrupt the comfortable environment of tumors, but it also has anti-fungal effect.

Best Alternative Treatment - Budwig Protocol

90% documented success in all types of Cancers

Bonding of Alpha-Linolenic Acid and Sulfurated Protein

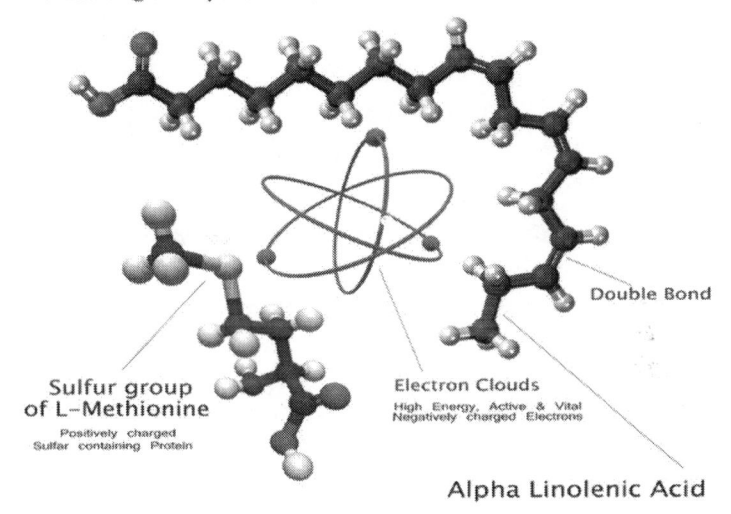

Sulfur group of L-Methionine
Positively charged Sulfar containing Protein

Electron Clouds
High Energy, Active & Vital Negatively charged Electrons

Double Bond

Alpha Linolenic Acid

Dr. Budwig has been referred to as a top European cancer research scientist, biochemist, pharmacologist, and physicist. Dr. Budwig was a seven-time Nobel Prize nominee.

In Germany in 1952, she was the central government's senior expert for fats and pharmaceutical drugs. She's considered one of the world's leading authorities on fats and oils. Her research has shown the tremendous effects that commercially processed fats and oils (having Trans fatty acids) have in destroying cell membranes and lowering the voltage in the cells of our bodies, which then result in chronic and terminal disease including cancer.

What we have forgotten is that we are body electric. The cells of our body fire electrically. They have a nucleus in the center of the cell which is positively charged, and the cell membrane, which is the outer lining of the cell, is negatively charged. We are all aware of how fats clog up our veins and arteries and are the leading cause of heart attacks, but we never looked beyond the end of our noses to see how these very dangerous fats and oils are affecting the overall health of our minds and bodies at the cellular level.

Dr. Budwig discovered that when unsaturated fats have been chemically treated, their unsaturated qualities are destroyed and the field of electrons removed. This commercial processing of fats destroys the field of electrons that the cell membranes (60-75 trillion cells) in our bodies must have to fire properly (i.e. function properly).

The fats' ability to associate with protein and thereby to achieve water solubility in the fluids of the living body is destroyed. As Budwig put it, "the battery is dead because the electrons in these fats and oils recharge it." When the electrons are destroyed the fats are no longer active and cannot flow into the capillaries and through the fine capillary networks. This is when circulation problems arise.

Without the proper metabolism of fats in our bodies, every vital function and every organ is affected. This includes the generation of new life and new cells. Our bodies produce over 500 million new cells daily. Dr. Budwig points out that in growing new cells, there is a polarity between the electrically positive nucleus and the electrically negative cell membrane with its high unsaturated fatty acids. During cell division, the cell, and new daughter cell must contain enough electron-rich fatty acids in the cell's surface area to divide off completely from the old cell. When this process is interrupted the body begins to die. In essence, these commercially processed fats and oils are shutting down the electrical field of the cells allowing chronic and terminal diseases to take hold of our bodies.

A very good example would be tumors. Dr. Budwig noted that "The formation of tumors usually happens as follows. In those body areas which normally host many growth processes, such as in the skin and membranes, the glandular organs, for example, the liver and pancreas or the glands in the stomach and intestinal tract—it is here that the growth processes are brought to a standstill. Because the polarity is missing, due to the lack of electron rich highly unsaturated fat, the course of growth is disturbed—the surface-active fats are not present; the substance becomes inactive before the maturing and shedding process of the cells ever takes place, which results in the formation of tumors."

She pointed out that this can be reversed by providing the simple foods, cottage cheese, and flax seed oil, which revises the stagnated growth processes. This naturally causes the tumor or tumors present to dissolve and the whole range of symptoms which indicate a "dead battery are cured." Dr. Budwig did not believe in the use of growth-inhibiting treatments such as chemotherapy or radiation. She was quoted as saying "I flat declare that the usual hospital treatments today, in a case of tumorous growth, most certainly leads to worsening of the disease or a speedier death, and in healthy people, quickly causes cancer."

Dr. Budwig discovered that when she combined flaxseed oil, with its powerful healing nature of essential electron rich unsaturated fats, and cottage cheese, which is rich in sulfur protein, the bonding produced makes the oil water soluble and easily absorbed into the cell membrane.

I found testimonials of people from around the world who had been diagnosed with terminal cancer (all types of cancer), sent home to die and were now living healthy, normal lives. Not only had Dr. Budwig been using her protocol for treating cancer in Europe, but she also treated other chronic diseases such as arthritis, heart infarction, irregular heartbeat, psoriasis, eczema (other skin diseases), immune deficiency syndromes (Multiple Sclerosis and other autoimmune diseases), diabetes, lungs (respiratory conditions), stomach ulcers, liver, prostate, strokes, brain tumors, brain (strengthens activity), arteriosclerosis and other chronic diseases. Dr. Budwig's protocol proved successful where orthodox traditional medicine was failing.

Prime Cause of Cancer

We are fighting with cancer since the dawn of history. Every year we discover new diagnostic modalities, better radiotherapy techniques and lots of new chemotherapy drugs. But we have completely failed to defeat this disease called cancer. Think again, are we really going on the right path? Does conventional Medicine really targets upon the prime cause of cancer???

Otto Warburg – Biography

Otto Heinrich Warburg (October 8, 1883 – August 1, 1970), son of physicist Emil Warburg, was a German physiologist, medical doctor and Nobel laureate. His mother was the daughter of a Protestant family of bankers and civil servants from Baden. Warburg studied chemistry under the great Emil Fischer, and earned his "Doctor of Chemistry" in Berlin in 1906. He then earned the degree of "Doctor of Medicine" in Heidelberg in 1911. Between 1908 and 1914, Warburg was affiliated with the Naples Marine Biological Station, in Naples, Italy, where he conducted research.

He served as an officer in the elite Uhlan (cavalry regiment) during the First World War, and was given the Iron Cross (1st Class) award for his bravery. Warburg is considered one of the 20th century's leading biochemists. Towards the end of the war, Albert Einstein, who had been a friend of Warburg's father Emil, wrote Warburg asking him to leave the army and return to academia, since it would be a tragedy for the world to lose his talents. Einstein and Warburg later became friends, and Einstein's work in physics had great influence on Otto's biochemical research.

While working at the Marine Biological Station, Warburg performed research on oxygen consumption in sea urchin eggs after fertilization, and proved that upon fertilization, the rate of respiration increases by as much as six fold. His experiments also proved that iron is essential for the development of the larval stage.

In 1918, Warburg was appointed professor at the Kaiser Wilhelm Institute for Biology in Berlin-Dahlem. By 1931 he was promoted as director of the Kaiser Wilhelm Institute for Cell Physiology, which was later on, renamed the Max Planck Society. Warburg investigated the metabolism of tumors and the respiration of cells, particularly cancer cells, and in 1931 was awarded the Nobel Prize in Physiology for his "discovery of the nature and mode of action of the respiratory enzyme."

Nomination for a second Nobel Prize

In 1944, Warburg was nominated for a second Nobel Prize in Physiology by Albert Szent-Györgyi, for his work on nicotinamide, the mechanism and enzymes involved in fermentation, and the discovery of flavin (in yellow enzymes), but was prevented from receiving it by Adolf Hitler's regime.

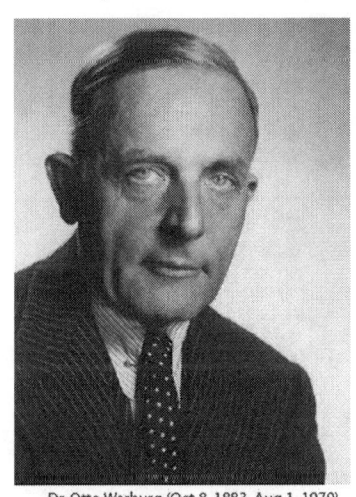

Otto Warburg edited and had much of his original work published in The Metabolism of Tumors and wrote New Methods of Cell Physiology (1962). Otto Warburg was thrilled when Oxford University awarded him an honorary doctorate.

In his later years, Warburg was convinced that illness is resulted from pollution; this caused him to become a bit of a health advocate. He insisted on eating bread made from wheat grown organically on his farm. When he visited restaurants, he often made arrangements to pay the full price for a cup of tea, but to only be served boiling water, from which he would make tea with a tea bag he had brought with him. He was also known to go to

Dr. Otto Warburg (Oct 8, 1883 Aug 1, 1970)

significant lengths to obtain organic butter, the quality of which he trusted.

The Otto Warburg Medal

The Otto Warburg Medal is intended to commemorate Warburg's outstanding achievements. It has been awarded by the German Society for Biochemistry and Molecular Biology since 1963. The prize honors and encourages pioneering achievements in fundamental biochemical and molecular biological research. The Otto Warburg Medal is regarded as the highest award for biochemists and molecular biologists in Germany.

Prime cause of Cancer

Warburg hypothesized that cancer growth is caused by tumor cells mainly generating energy (as e.g. adenosine triphosphate / ATP) by anaerobic breakdown of glucose (known as fermentation, or anaerobic respiration). This is in contrast to healthy cells, which mainly generate energy from oxidative breakdown of pyruvate. Pyruvate is an end product of glycolysis, and is oxidized within the mitochondria. Hence, and according to Warburg, cancer should be interpreted as a mitochondrial dysfunction.

In short, Warburg summarized that all normal cells absolutely require oxygen, but cancer cells can live without oxygen - a rule without exception. Deprive a cell 35% of its oxygen for 48 hours and it would become cancerous. **Dr. Otto Warburg clearly mentioned that the root cause of cancer is lack of oxygen in the cells.**

He also discovered that cancer cells are anaerobic (do not breathe oxygen), get the energy by fermenting glucose and produce levo-rotating lactic acid, and the body becomes acidic. Cancer cannot survive in the presence of high levels of oxygen, as found in an alkaline state.

He postulated that sulfur containing protein and some unknown fat is required to attract oxygen into the cell. This fat plays a major role in the respiration and functioning of Warburg respiratory enzyme. He thought it would be butyric acid and made experiment, but this attempt was a failure. For many decades scientists were trying to identify this unknown and mysterious fat but nobody succeeded (Otto Warburg, Wikipedia).

Dr. Johanna Budwig - Biography & Science

Birth of an angel

A lovely couple, Hermann Budwig and Elisabeth, lived in Essen town of Germany situated on the bank of river Ruhr. On the eve of 30th September, 1908 Elisabeth delivered a brilliant and lucky angel. Hermann and Elisabeth were very happy, and celebrating. They called her Johanna. In German, Johanna means a gift from God. In the family and neighborhood everybody was talking that Johanna is very lucky, she will study in a college and become a big doctor. Actually, 1908 was very fortunate and important year for the freedom of women in Germany. Government for the first time in history, changed laws, and allowed women to study in college and Universities. Also the German parliament passed a legislation to allow women to become members of political parties and prestigious clubs. Though women were given new rights and freedom, liberalization was slow and old values still persisted.

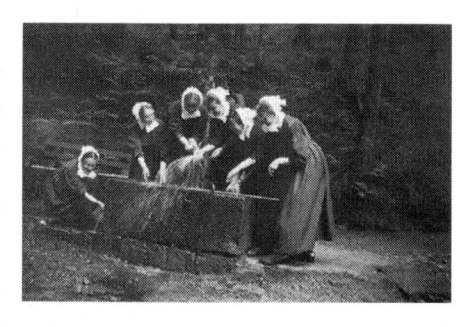

The tough life of a sage of science

Unluckily, Elisabeth died in 1920; family members thought that her father, being a poor loco mechanic, might not look after Johanna. So she was sent to an orphanage. This was a great shock for the little Johanna, but it had one positive side also. Education up to higher level was totally free for orphans.

In 1926, Germany was slowly recovering from the after effects of the First World War. Economic conditions were improving. Scholars and scientists were developing new technologies in every field. One third of all Nobel Prizes were being given to German academics.

Deaconess at Kaiserswerth

Johanna was very intelligent and sharp in studies from the beginning. In order to achieve good future, she decided to join the renowned Deaconess's Institute of Kaiserswerth in 1925. Theodor Fliedner, a pastor, founded Kaiserswerth Institute for welfare of unmarried mothers, prisoners, patients, orphans and poor children in 1836. In the beginning a Hospital and a Nursing School was established. This school was very famous Nursing School of that time. Florence Nightingale, known as mother of modern nursing, also studied in this Deaconess School in 1850. Intelligent Johanna easily got admission in this Institute. She was made a "deaconess" on March 30, 1932. This was the most appropriate place for her. There was a 1000 bedded hospital, pharmacy and a boarding school. She decided to study pharmacy.

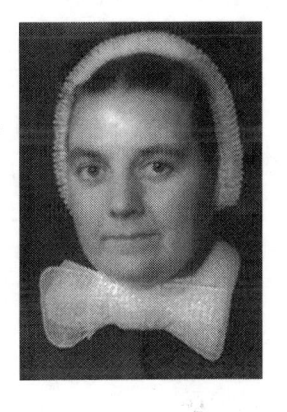

After completing preliminary education in Kaiserswerth, she joined Münster University for further studies. Her analytical thinking and precise knowledge was noticed by her Professor Dr Hans Paul Kaufmann. He always encouraged and helped her. Here she passed state examination in pharmacy and was rewarded distinction in chemistry in 1936. Then she continued further education in physics, and received the title "Doctor of Science" at the University of Münster in 1938. On August 1, 1939, she was appointed as in-charge of pharmacy at the Military Hospital in Kaiserswerth.

Next month, Hitler's military forces attacked Poland. During war time, brave Johanna was busy in organizing and expanding the pharmacy. The war was not an easy time. There were two thousand people living in Kaiserswerth. Johanna was responsible for ensuring that there were enough medicines in this time of rationing and a thriving black market. She was well prepared and ready to fulfill any emergency demand for her patients. Many of her fellow deaconesses were often jealous and not co-operating but she continued evolving her professional skills. She was strong and was confronting every opponent (Dr. Johanna Budwig Stiftung).

Dr Budwig's scientific thinking, work and career

After Second World War, Johanna left Kaiserswerth in 1949. Soon Prof. Kaufmann came to know that she had left Kaiserswerth. He immediately met and persuaded her to work with him in Münster University, as he was always impressed from her talent. He converted the basement of his house into a laboratory and arranged all facilities for her research. He was famous as Fat Pope in the whole Europe.

On Prof. Kaufmann's recommendation, Johanna was appointed as the chief expert for drugs and fats at the Federal Institute for Fats Research, Germany. This was the country's largest office issuing the approval of new drugs used for cancer. Many applications had been submitted to her for approval. These were the medications for cancer therapy with the sulfhydryl group (sulfur-containing protein compounds). Everywhere she saw that fats played a role in cellular respiration, also in expert reports provided by well-known professors like Prof. Nonnenbruch. Unfortunately, fats could only be detected in the late stage, and there were no method to distinguish between fats chemically.

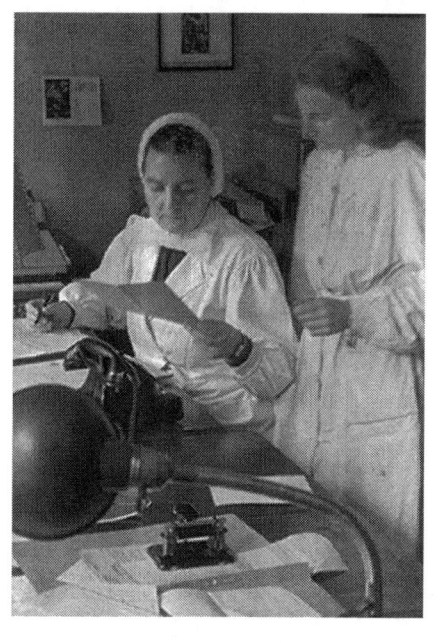

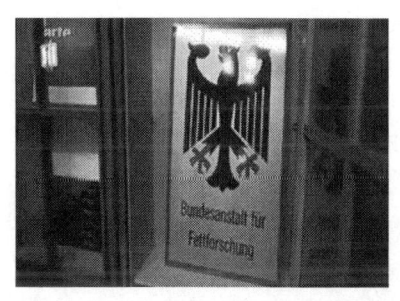

By this time, she developed paper chromatography. With this technique for first time she was able to detect fatty acids and lipoproteins directly even in 0.1 ml of blood. She used Co60 isotopes successfully to produce the first differential reaction for fatty acids, and produced the first direct iodine value via radioiodine. She also developed control of atmosphere in a closed system by using gas systems which act as antioxidants. She further developed Coloring methods, separating effects of fats and fatty acids. She too studied their behavior in blue and red light with fluorescent dyes.

Using rhodamine red dye, she studied the electrical behavior of the unsaturated fatty acids with their "halo". With this technique she could prove that electron rich highly unsaturated Linoleic and Linolenic fatty acids (Flax oil being the richest source) were the mysterious and undiscovered decisive fats required to attract oxygen into the cells, which Otto Warburg could not find. She studied the electromagnetic function of pi-electrons of the linolenic acid in the cell membranes, for nerve function, secretions, mitosis, as well as cell division. She also examined the synergism of the sulfur containing protein with the pi-electrons of the highly unsaturated fatty acids and their significance for the formation of the hydrogen bridge between fat and protein, which represent "the only path" for fast and focused Transport of electrons during respiration. This research was extensively published in 1950 in Neue Wege in der Fettforschung (New Directions in Fat Research) and other publications.

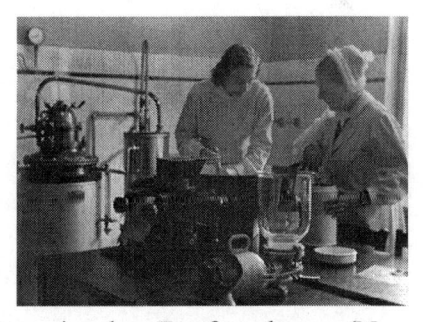

This immediately caused an excitement and turmoil in the scientific community. Everybody thought that it would open new doors in Cancer research. She also proved that hydrogenated fats and refined oils including all Trans-fatty acids were not having vital electrons and were respiratory poisons.

During her research, she found that the blood of seriously ill cancer patients had deficiency of unsaturated essential fats (Linoleic and Linolenic fatty acids), lipoproteins, phosphatides, and hemoglobin. She also had noticed that cancer patients had a strange greenish-yellow substance in their blood which is not present in the blood of healthy people (Budwig, Cancer The Problem And The Solution).

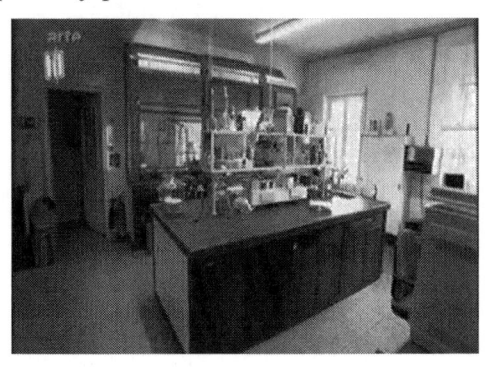

She wanted to develop a healing program for cancer. So she enrolled over 642 cancer patients from four hospitals in Münster. She gave Flax oil and Cottage Cheeseto these patients. After just three months, patients began to improve in health and strength, the yellow green substance in their blood began to disappear, tumors gradually receded and at the same time the nutrients began to rise.

This way she developed a simple cure for cancer, based on the consumption of Flax oil with low fat Quark or cottage cheese, raw organic diet, mild exercise, Flax oil massage and the healing powers of the sun. It was a great victory and the first milestone in the battle against cancer. She treated approx. 2500 cancer patients during last few decades. Prof. Halme of surgery clinic in Helsinki used to keep records of her patients. According to him her success was over 90%, and this was achieved in cases, which were rejected by Allopathic doctors.

Dr. Budwig was a courageous scientist. She **loudly and convincingly argued that consumption of highly processed foods, particularly edible oils and margarines, which block the oxidation processes in the cells, are responsible for the development of cancer and other degenerative diseases.** She met with great resistance from food industry giants, who were doing everything to prevent the spread of her sensational discovery. In 1952, under the influence of strong pressure from this lobby, she lost her job and was barred from the research work.

Joins Medical School at Göttingen

Opponents of Dr. Johanna blamed her that she should not treat cancer patients because she doesn't have a doctor's degree. She felt this and eventually joined medical school in Göttingen in 1955. Budwig was 47 years old at that time. She also continued her research work along with her studies. *Budwig successfully treated Prof. Martius's wife, who suffered from Breast Cancer*

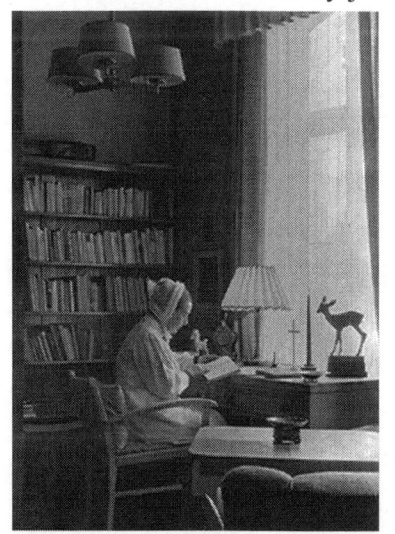

One night a woman came with her small child whose arm was supposed to be amputated due to a tumor. She treated her and soon the amputation surgery was dismissed, and the child quickly did very well.

A Swiss woman came to her clinic in Göttingen. She suffered from Colon Cancer with metastasis and intestinal obstruction. Several doctors examined her, and were to be operated on Christmas Eve. On Budwig's request, she was treated by her protocol. The tumor of the colon quickly subsided. Seven weeks later, she was discharged without any detectable tumor. It is interesting that the Swiss custom officer was not ready to believe that the submitted passport belonged to same lady. Her look was so much changed! At home her daughter welcomed saying: "You look healthy, younger and more beautiful (from her book The Death of the Tumor – Vol. II).

After this, University allowed her to treat cancer patients with her oil-protein diet. She was getting miraculous results. University professors were excited with the results, but wanted that she should also include chemo and radiotherapy. She was rigid and didn't want to compromise. So she had differences and conflicts with her professors and ultimately left Göttingen (Budwig, Cancer The Problem And The Solution).

Last Destination - Dietersweiler-Freudenstadt

Eventually, she shifted to Dietersweiler-Freudenstadt, where she lived till her death. There she completed Ph.D. in Naturopathy so that she could legally treat cancer patients. She continued treating her patients in Freudenstadt. In 1968 she created unique Eldi oils for massage and enema, called Electron Differential Oils after performing precise spectroscopic measurements of the light absorption in different oils. *US pain institute has written somewhere: "What this crazy woman does with her ELDI oils, none of us manages to do via pain killers."*

Budwig conducted more than 200 lectures worldwide. Dr. Budwig was popular in the U.S. as FLAX SEED lady from Freudenstadt. She delivered her last public Lecture in Freudenstadt on March 3, 1999. On November 28, 2002, she fell down in her bathroom and got a fracture in right femur neck. She was admitted in a nursing home and ultimately died on May 19, 2003.

Budwig Protocol

The Budwig Protocol is one of the most widely followed alternative treatments for cancer and other diseases. The diet seems simple, but foods are powerful and can heal a person.

Transition Diet

The Transition diet is especially recommended for patients of liver, pancreatic or gall bladder cancers. The basic principle is that for 3 days nothing is eaten and drunk except the following written and at least three times daily warm tea (herbal teas from peppermint, rose hip, mallow or green tea) is drunk. Dr Budwig has recommended variant 1 for patients with a relatively good energy state, and variant 2 and 3 mainly for seriously ill patients.

Variant 1

Variant 1 for three days, 250 g of linomel or alternatively freshly crushed Flax seed is eaten together with the following:
- Freshly pressed fruit juices without added sugar.
- Freshly pressed vegetable juices such as carrot, celery juice, red beetroots and apple juice.
- Chinese tea and black tea are allowed in the morning
- Honey for sweetening is allowed. Just as grape juice for drinking and as a sweetener. Energetically weak patients can also consume sparkling wine and linomel.

Variant 2

For three days, oat meal cereal very hour with linomel is eaten daily with the following juices:
- Freshly pressed fruit juices or freshly pressed vegetable juices such as carrot, celery juice, beetroot and apple juice.
- Chinese tea and black tea are allowed in the morning.
- Honey for sweetening is allowed. Just as grape juice for drinking and as a sweetener.

- Energetically weak patients can also consume sparkling wine and linomel.

Variant 3

For three days, oatmeal soup with linomel is given three times a day together with the following juices:
- Freshly pressed fruit juices or fruit juices without added sugar.
- Freshly pressed vegetable juices such as carrot, celery juice, beetroot and apple juice.
- Chinese tea and black tea are allowed in the morning.
- Honey for sweetening is allowed. Just as grape juice for drinking and as a sweetener.
- Energetically weak patients can also consume sparkling wine and linomel.

It is often experienced frequently that patients mixed all three variants and "nevertheless" had good results. So better you to stick to one variant. (Budwig – Cancer The Problem And The Solution 2005: p.36).

Budwig Diet

The Budwig Protocol is necessary for many diseases from cancer to type 2 diabetes and heart disease to autoimmune diseases, etc. Its purpose is to energize the cells by restoring the natural electrical potential in the cell. Many human diseases are caused by "sick cells" which have lost their normal electrical potential; generally via a lower ATP energy in the cell's mitochondria.

6:00 AM – Sauerkraut juice

A glass of sauerkraut juice consumed before breakfast every morning. It is rich in vitamins including C, enzymes and helps develop the health-promoting gut flora. Sauerkraut is cabbage that has been pickled by natural fermentation, mainly with lactobacillus bacteria. It is slightly salty, sharp and sour. Well made, it is much nicer than it sounds. You may also consume another glass of sauerkraut juice later in the day.

It interesting that sauerkraut contains right rotating lactic acids and is highly alkaline and neutralizes levo-rotating lactic acids and makes our body alkaline. That is why Marcus Porcius Cato the Elder issued a statement - Carcinomas are incurable except with the treatment with Sauerkraut.

8:00 AM Breakfast

Green or herbal tea

Start breakfast with a cup of warm herbal or green tea. Sweeten with only natural honey. You can add lemon or grape juice. Patient should take such a tea before or with Linomel Muesli. You may consume 4-5 such teas in a day.

Linomel Muesli or Oil-Protein Muesli

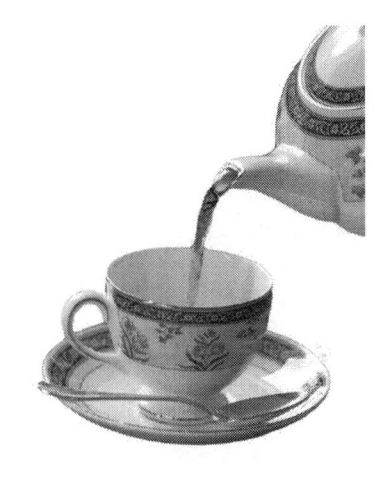

This should be made fresh and consumed within 15 minutes. It is full of high energy pi-electrons, attract oxygen in the cells and capable of healing cell membranes. It is full of energy-rich omega-3 fats, has power to attract healing photons from sun through resonance. As "Om" is divine word and synonym of God in India. According to Hindu Mythology, the whole universe is located inside "Om", so the name Omkhand has been given to this wonderful recipe in Hindi.

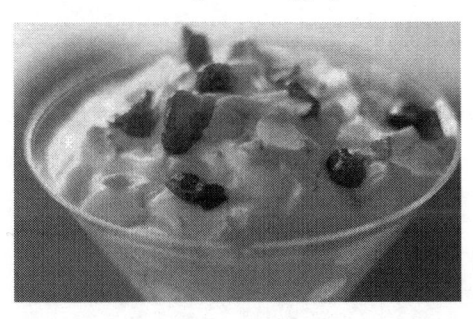

Ingredients

- 3 Tbsp cold pressed organic Flax seed oil (FO)
- 100-125gm (6 Tbsp) Quark or Cottage Cheese(CC)

- 2 Tbsp freshly ground Flax seeds
- 2 Tbsp milk
- 1 cup fruits
- ¼ cup dried nuts
- Natural honey
- Flavorings – lemon, apple cider vinegar, cinnamon, pure cacao, natural vanilla, shredded coconut etc.

Recipe

Place 2 tablespoons Linomel or freshly ground Flax seeds in a small bowl. It is covered with raw, crushed or diced seasonal fruits depending on the season. Pour some orange or grape juice over this. Linomel^{Tm} is a brand name and originally created and patented by Budwig. It is a cereal made from cracked Flax Seed, a small amount of honey and a little milk powder.

Then the Quark-Flax seed oil cream is prepared in as follows: First add Flax seed oil, milk and honey and blend briefly with a hand-held immersion electric blender, then gradually add the Quark in smaller portions. Blend till oil and Quark is thoroughly mixed with no separated oil. Then it is seasoned differently everyday with different flavorings such as vanilla, cinnamon or various fruits such as banana, apple, lemon, orange juice, or berries.

Use various fruits such as fresh berries, apple, cherry, orange, banana, papaya, grapes etc. Add other fresh fruit if you like, totaling ½ to 1 cup of fruit. Budwig specially advised to use berries like strawberry, blueberry, raspberry, cheery etc. because berries have ellagic acids which are strong cancer fighters.

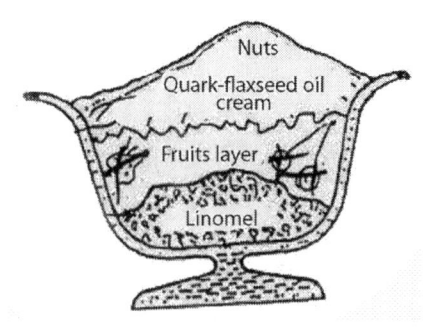

Add organic raw nuts such as walnuts, almonds, raisins or Brazil nuts. They have sulfurated proteins, omega-3 fats and vitamins. Brazil nut is especially important because a single nut provides you with all of the selenium you need for the day. Selenium is very important to boost immune power. Peanuts are prohibited.

For variety and flavor, try natural vanilla, cinnamon, lemon juice, pure cocoa or shredded coconut.

Once blended in Budwig Cream, Quark and Flax seed oil form a new substance called lipoprotein. Lipoprotein is a water soluble complex. The Quark is rich in the sulfur-containing amino acids, methionine and cysteine. These positively charged amino acids attract the negatively charged electron clouds in fatty acid chains and exhibit a stabilizing effect on the highly unsaturated, otherwise easily oxidized fats. Thus, the amino acids protect the polyunsaturated fatty acids from the Flax seed oil against oxidation which, as a result, are able to enter the human body unchanged and with their full energy potential. The result: they are much more valuable to cells and their membranes. Consequently, one could say that Quark excels as a protector for the polyunsaturated fatty acids.

Sulfur-rich amino acids play a wealth of roles in many vital functions in our bodies. In combination with polyunsaturated fatty acids, they are important partners in regulating the uptake of oxygen and its utilization by the cell. They therefore contribute significantly to a strong immune system, healthy metabolism, and mental vitality. For many generations, people have been getting their omega-3 fatty acids from fish, vegetables, nuts, and seeds. Our health literally depends on the regular consumption of the essential omega-3 and omega-6 fatty acids, alpha-linolenic acid (ALA) and linoleic acid (LA). Our bodies require these fatty acids in order to synthesize their cell membranes as well as for a variety of metabolic processes and heal the cancer and other diseases.

Tips for making the Budwig Mixture
- Follow directions properly! It is important to add things to the mixture in the right order. If you mix them in the

wrong order you may lose a lot of the opportunity to convert the oil-soluble omega-3 into water soluble-omega-3.
- Keep the Flax seed oil refrigerated.
- Immersion blender is a must.
- The mixture can be flavored differently every day by adding nuts and fruits preferably organic such as pecans, almonds or walnuts (not peanuts), banana, organic cocoa, shredded coconut, pineapple (fresh) blueberries, raspberries, cinnamon, vanilla or (freshly) squeezed fruit juice.
- Consume immediately for best results.

10 AM Vegetable juice

Freshly squeezed vegetable juice from carrots, beets, celery, tomato, and radish, lemon as well as green vegetables - stinging nettle, lettuce or spinach. Apple is added to sweeten and enhance the taste. Carrot & beet juices are especially helpful to the liver and have strong cancer fighting properties. Vary vegetables. Some tasty and nutritious combinations are beet and apple juice, carrot and apple, carrot and beet, asparagus and apple, celery and apple, celery and carrot. Beet juice should not be taken alone. If taken alone it may cause red or pink urine (beeturia).

She also frequently recommended the following juices:

1. Nettle juice - Especially in the spring, Dr Budwig recommended to puree nettles with water and a lemon.

2. Radish juice - For this, a radish is first crushed and then thrown together with a lemon into the juicer. This juice is by the way durable for several days and Dr Budwig has sometimes recommended her patients to drink a small quantity of them every day.

3. Coltsfoot juice - For this juice, with the exception of the harder old rootstock, the entire remaining underground shoot is mixed with a few flowers and some milk and honey.

4. Horseradish juice - Mix 3-5 cm horseradish together with an apple and (raw) milk. Depending on the quantity of milk you can change the taste. Dr Budwig recommended this juice above all to workmen and to stimulate the appetite. Freshly pressed means, by the way, that you drink the juice within 5 minutes after pressing. In some cases, Dr Budwig prescribed a second juice 30 to 60 minutes later.

12:15 PM Lunch

Salad Platter: Salad plate with homemade cottage cheese-Flax seed mayonnaise. As salad also use: dandelion, cress, celery, tomato, cucumber, lettuce, radish, cabbage, broccoli, green horseradish and pepper.

Delicious mayo salad dressing can be prepared by mixing together 2 Tbsp (30 ml) Flax Oil, 2 Tbsp (30 ml) milk, and 2 Tbsp (30 ml) cottage cheese. Then add 2 tablespoons (30 ml) of Lemon juice (or Apple Cider Vinegar) and add 1 teaspoon (2.5 g) Mustard powder plus some herbs of your choice. Other alternative dressing can be made by mixing Flax Oil, lemon juice, Mustard and some herbs (Budwig, The Oil-Protein Diet Cookbook, 1994).

Main Course: Vegetables cooked in water, then flavored with Oleolox and herbs possibly with oatmeal, soy sauce, curry etc. Vegetable broth flavored with a little Oleolox and yeast flakes. As side dish for the vegetables: buckwheat, brown rice, millet or potatoes can be used. One or two slices of Ezekiel bread can be taken. Use lot of dried fruits in the main meal also.

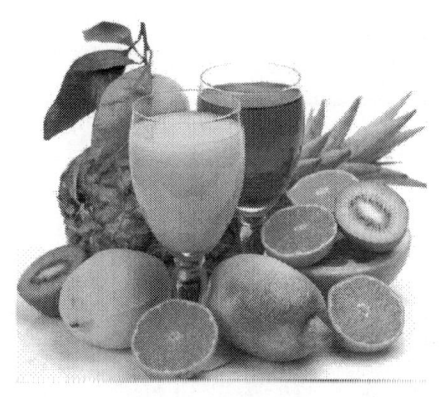

Lunch Dessert: Cottage cheese/ Flax oil mixture served as a dessert, prepared with dry fruits and fruits such as apple, or poured over a fruit salad. You already know how to prepare it perfectly. You will find wonderful recipes for a delicious dessert in the Oil-Protein cookbook by Budwig. Please note that the dessert is **"a must"** and should definitely be eaten. So keep your main course light so you may enjoy the dessert happily.

The form of preparation as "fruit foam," "Linovita" or "red coat in the snow" (in Oil-Protein cookbook) is always welcoming for the healthy and the sick. In all the gimmicks in the preparation of the delicious desserts, one should be aware: Quark and Flaxseed give the patient immense power within a short space of time. Always fresh and beautiful, always freshly interesting, this important food for life should be for the sick and for the whole family.

3 PM Fruit juices

In the afternoon, Dr Budwig recommended different kinds of fruit juices e.g. apples, grapes, cherries, pineapples, papaya, or apricot, sparkling wine or wine - with or without Flaxseeds or with or without a few drops Flaxseed oil.

Budwig preferred papaya juice and recommended her patients to drink at least every 2 days a glass of papaya juice. The main reason for this was definitely the protein splitting enzyme papain.

6 PM Dinner

The evening meal should be light and served early, around 6 p.m. A warm meal may be prepared using brown rice, buckwheat or oat meal. Never consume corn or soy beans. Dishes made with buckwheat grouts are most easily tolerated and nourishing. Use only honey to sweeten. Soup or more solid dishes can be combined with a tasty sauce according to preference. Use OLEOLOX liberally also to sweet sauces and soups, making them nourishing and a richer source of energy.

8:30 PM

A glass of organic red wine may be consumed. All things are a matter of correct dosage. This glass of red wine is not a "must" program. In fact, seriously ill patients having pain and discomfort just starting on the oil-protein diet, it is recommended to serve a glass of red wine mixed with freshly ground Flax seeds to tide them over while going off pain killers (Budwig, Cancer The Problem And The Solution).

METRIC CONVERSION TABLE	
10 g = 0.35 oz	5 cc = 1 teaspoon
100 g = 3.5 oz	15 cc = 1 tablespoon
150 g = 5.25 oz	30 cc = 1 ounce
250 g = 8.8 oz	250 cc = 1 cup
454 g = 1 lb	960 cc = 1 qt
Oz = ounce lb = pound qt = quart Tsp = teaspoon Tbsp = tablespoon	

Precautions

Drink filtered water - Use RO (Reverse Osmosis) water for drinking, cooking and enemas.

Eat Organic Diet - Always try to eat organic food.

Dental Care –

Mercury is a Carcinogenic as well as a Poison! The root canals of dead teeth are full of bacteria that attack the liver and lymphatic system. From Amalgam fillings the mercury slowly leaks out of the filings. The ADA cleverly defends the use of amalgam in spite of the fact that there is sufficient evidence that patients with many severe problems, including psychotic episodes and fatal allergic reactions, were just cured by removing the amalgam. It is advisable to rather have a ceramic filling than be slowly poisoned by mercury. Even gold filling is dangerous; it acts as battery producing electrical current. Be informed that the effect of drugs, including poison, is dose dependant and cumulative.

Fluoride is not only toxic but it is also carcinogenic. Fluoride has never been proven to prevent tooth decay. It has been outlawed in many countries or groups of countries because the evidence is overwhelming that fluoride causes premature aging, so drink bottled water and use fluoride-free toothpaste (American Cancer Institute - 1963).

I highly recommend helping you avoid fillings in the first place. Holistic dentist recommend 3% H_2O_2 as a gargle or rinse, or making a paste using baking soda. H_2O_2 usage three times a day is advised. It is great for cleaning dentures, too.

Frying and deep frying - Frying and deep frying is not allowed to cook patient's food. Never heat any oil in the kitchen. By heating oils the wealth of high energy electrons is destroyed and Trans fats and dangerous toxic chemicals such as acrylamides are formed in the oil. Boiling and steaming are good practices. You can fry vegetables etc. in water and add oleolox before serving. Water is the safest medium for frying, says Lothar Hirneise.

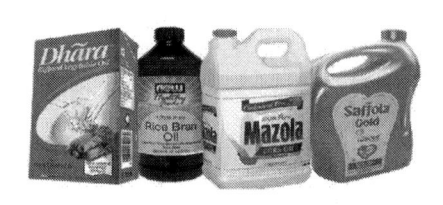

Chemo and Radio -

Chemotherapy is aimed at destruction of the tumor, and it destroys many living cells, and the entire person. Anything that disturbs growth is fatal because growth is an elementary function of life. We cannot achieve something good with bad tools.

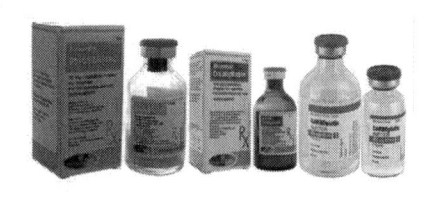

Dr. Budwig rejects Chemo and Radiation Therapy. Budwig used to say with full confidence and clarity, "My treatment targets on the real cause of cancer; it fills cancer cells with high energy pi-electrons and attracts oxygen into the cells. And cancer cells start to breathe and produce vital energy."

Man-made Supplements - With this treatment man-made antioxidants, synthetic vitamins and pain killers should not be given. The dose of anticoagulants and aspirin should be adjusted by your doctor. Dr. Budwig favors natural, herbal and homeopathy instead of man-made and synthetic supplements, vitamins and pain killers (Budwig, Cancer The Problem And The Solution).

Prohibitions of Budwig Protocol

In this protocol there are certain restrictions. They are as important as the diet itself. It is very difficult to defeat the cancer without strictly following these rules.

Sugar is strictly forbidden

Sugar, Jiggery, molasses, maple syrup and artificial sweeteners like xylitol, aspartame are not permitted. You can use only natural honey, stevia and fruit juices – all off course unprocessed.

Avoid meats, eggs and fish

Meat, fish, poultry, eggs, and butter are never allowed. Preserved meat is like a poison. It is highly processed and treated with dangerous antibiotics, preservatives and nitrates.

Stop using Hydrogenated Fat and Refined oil

You can never eat pizza, burger, fast food, fried food, biscuits etc. as they all are made by hydrogenated margarine and shortenings. Hydrogenation is a very dangerous process, used to increase shelf life of fats. In this process (oil is heated at very high temperature and hydrogen is passed through oils in presence of nickel) killing Trans fats are formed, high energy live and vital electrons are destroyed and nutrients are damaged. Hydrogenated Fats is just a dead, nutrition-less and cancer causing liquid plastic. Budwig always preached against these damaging fats. She has allowed low fat cheese, oleolox and coconut oil.

Preservatives and Processed Food

You should not eat Potato chips, soft drinks etc. which are full of preservatives. Never consume highly processed food e.g. ready to eat packed foods, pasta, pastries, bread and soy products, tofu etc. However good quality soy souse is permitted.

Microwave, Teflon, Aluminum and Plastic

Never cook in microwave oven. Food cooked in microwave become toxic and deformed. Also don't use aluminum, plastic, Teflon coated cookware and aluminum foils. Use stainless steel, iron, china clay or glass utensils instead.

Chemicals and pesticides are not allowed

Avoid pesticides and chemicals, even those in household products & cosmetics. Stay away from mosquito repellants, sun screen lotions and sun glasses.

Wear natural fibers

Don't wear clothes made using synthetic fiber like nylon, polyester and acrylic. Budwig put great emphasis on the fact that her patients only wore natural fabrics such as cotton or satin, since they too can influence the magnetic field of our body.

Bed

Don't use on foam pillow and mattress. She recommended horsehair mattresses. Latex mattresses are the second choice. In any case, however, you should always replace mattresses that have metal spring cores.

CRT TV and mobile phones

These emit dangerous electromagnetic radiation, so do not use them. You can watch LCD and plasma TVs.

No left over

Food should be prepared fresh and eaten soon after preparation to maximize intake of health giving electrons and enzymes (Budwig, Cancer The Problem And The Solution).

Few Desserts recipes by Dr. Budwig

Fujiya delight

Ingredients for 3 people:
250 cc grape juice, 250 cc pure currant juice,
8g agar-agar, Quark-Flaxseed oil,
Milk, honey, vanilla cream

Preparation:
Heat the grape juice till it boils, then add the currant juice, agar-agar, stirring constantly for 5 minutes, and allow to cool. Now divide this mass to 3 narrow, tall cups, which have been rinsed with cold water. It is preferable if these cups have a bottom diameter of only 3- 4 cm. Refrigerate to cool. Now mix a Quark-Flaxseed oil cream with milk, honey and vanilla. Turn the red jelly upside down onto glass plates. The Quark-Flaxseed oil cream is placed on the top so that only the upper half is covered with the Quark-Flaxseed oil cream, so that top looks like the Snow caped Mount Fujiyama.

(The beautiful hotel with a gorgeous view of the Fujiyama is called "Fujiya", hence the dessert "Fujiya".)

Linovita-in-love in wine jelly

Ingredients: for 5 people:
250 cc of grape juice, 250 ccm of white wine,
8 agar-agar, 4 tablespoons of milk,
8 tablespoons of Flaxseed oil, 2 teaspoons of honey,
200-250 g of Quark, 2 liqueur glasses
Vodka, plum (Slibowitz) or cherry brandy or rum

Preparation:
The wine jelly is prepared by heating 250 cc of grape juice till it boils. Agar-agar is stirred with a little wine and placed in the boiling grape juice. Immediately remove from the cooking plate and add the remaining wine gradually with constant stirring.

After about 5 minutes, the jelly mixture clears itself. You can now divide to approx. 5 glass bowls or champagne glasses. Immediately afterwards, mix the Quark-Flaxseed oil cream from Flaxseed oil, milk, honey and Quark. Finally, add 2 liqueur glasses of vodka or slibovitz or cherry brandy or rum into the Quark-Flaxseed oil cream. This Quark-Flaxseed oil mixture is evenly divided on the ready to-use bowls so that the Quark-Flaxseed oil cream partly sinks down in the middle. It is served after complete solidification.

Ice cream with cocoa

Ingredients:
  3 tablespoons of Flaxseed oil, 3 tablespoons of milk,
  1 tablespoon of honey, 100g of Quark, 100 g of hazelnuts,
  2 tablespoons of cocoa

Preparation:
Quark, Flaxseed oil, milk and honey are mixed in the blender, then the hazelnuts are added, well blended and finally, cocoa is added to the mixture. Now pour the entire mixture into the ice-maker and place it in the fridge compartment of the refrigerator. This mixture with a nougat flavor gives the various combinations mentioned here the dark color contrast. For very ill people these preparations are very important, especially when there is a general lack of appetite.

*(*Oil-Protein Diet by Lothar Hirneise *available at http://www.hirneise.com/page-8/page-19/)*

ELDI oils

Dr. Budwig created unique ELDI oils, called electron differential oils after performing precise spectroscopic measurements of the light absorption in different oils - specifying that the oils contained pi-electron clouds from Flax oil, wheat germ oil plus vitamin-E in its natural complex, etheric oils and sulfhydryl groups.

Dr. Johanna Budwig said, "The sun is my preferred treatment modality, as is ELDI oil, used externally to stimulate the absorption of the long-wave band of the sun. I have used ELDI oils extensively since 1968 for body massage as well as in the selective application of oil packs. US pain institute has written somewhere: "What this crazy woman does with her ELDI oils, none of us manages to do via pain killers." Dr. Budwig has mentioned that if ELDI oil is not available, you may use Flax oil instead. *You can buy ELDI oils at: www.sensei.de*

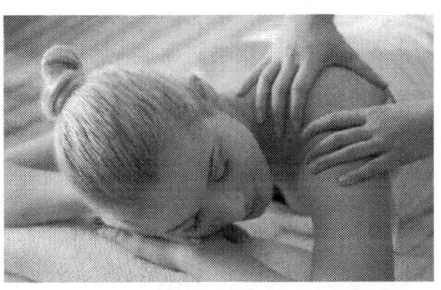

Massage Benefits

- Since ancient time massage has been part of cancer healing. Think of your lymphatics as a trash-disposal system for your body. Massage initiates lymphatic drainage, you push the trash out of your body and you're helping your immune system.
- Massage therapy is sometimes the first really pleasant touch a patient is able to experience.
- Massage also releases endorphins (our body's natural painkillers), stimulates lymph movement, and stretches tissues throughout the body. It's energizing, stimulating, and pretty good feeling.

ELDI oil plans:

A: For cancer patients in support of the energy level
1. Full-body rubbings in the morning
2. ELDI oil R enema with 200ml every 2-3 days
3. Wrap at the "place of the happening"

B: For energetically weak patients
1. Full-body rubbings in the morning and in the evening
2. Enema: standard plan for ELDI oil R
3. Wrap at the "place of the happening"
4. Daily liver wrap with ELDI oil sage

Additional information:
- Make sure that you make once a week an (deep/high) enema with water or coffee.
- If you make daily coffee enemas, then start in the morning with the coffee enema and then with the ELDI R enema, but only if your energetic level allows you to make two enemas daily. Otherwise, only make the ELDI R enema. (Oil Protein Diet by Lothar Hirneise)

ELDI oils from SENSEI (www.sensei.de) are produced in a permanent cold chain in a European oil mill and marketed under the name of Electron Differentiation Oils. There are two qualities. A 6-star organic quality and a 5-star quality, which are produced exclusively for the IOPDF (www.iopdf.com).

Cost factor ELDI oils

Again and again we hear that for reasons of cost, patients use Flax seed oil instead of ELDI oil R for an enema. Please do not do so, because Flax seed oil does not react in the same way as ELDI oil R. Instead, use cheap ELDI oils from IOPDF or reduce the amount of oil.

Procedure –

Two times a day, i.e. morning and evening, rub ELDI Oil or Flax oil into the skin over the whole body, a bit more intensely on the shoulders, armpits and groin area (where plenty of lymphatic vessels are present) as well as the problem areas, such as the breast, stomach, liver, etc. Leave the oil on the skin for about 20 minutes and follow with a warm water shower without washing with soap. After 10 minutes take another shower, this time using a mild soap, and then relax for 15-20 minutes.

Once the body has been oiled and the ELDI Oil or Flax oil has penetrated the skin, the warm water will open the skin pores and the oil penetrates the skin more deeply. The second shower, where one washes with soap, cleanses the skin so that clothes and linen will not become overly soiled.

Oil Packs

Take a piece of cloth made of pure cotton. Cut to a size to fit the body part, such as the knee. Soak the cotton cloth with oil, place on the knee etc., cover it with a piece of polythene and wrap it up with an elastic bandage. Leave overnight. Remove in the morning and wash the knee; repeat in the evening. Keep applying the same procedure for weeks, you get good results. You also use Flax oil or castor oil for these local applications if you do not get ELDI oils . Dr Budwig generally recommended ELDI sage and should be used in the following indications:

- Tumors
- Painful skin areas
- Metastases
- Hepatic impairment and liver support
- Kidney problems
- Bladder disorders
- Intestinal cramps
- Lung disorders
- Bone disorders of all kinds

ELDI Oil Enema

Enemas are used in the Oil-Protein Diet exclusively for the energy intake and not for the purification of the intestine. Dr Budwig used to give ELDI oil or Flax oil enema to her serious patients. Budwig used to get immediate and miraculous results with the most seriously ill patients. Flax seed Oil enema also give similar results.

I recommend you to make the first enemas only with 100ml and then increase over several days to 250ml. Some patients have enemas with 500ml oil and positively reported on it. 500ml are however the absolute exception and mostly not necessary. Usually 250ml suffice.

Incidentally, smaller amounts are also easily introduced with an enema syringe instead of with an enema bucket. Enema syringes are available in sizes up to 350ml and are easy to handle.

Standard plan for ELDI oil R: Day 1 = 100ml, day 2 = 100ml, day 3 = 150ml, day 4 = 150ml, day 5 = 200ml, day 6 = 200ml and day 7 = 250ml.

From the seventh day, one remains at 250ml, and so long until the patient is significantly better. Then you can go back to 100ml - 150ml, always together with 1-2 daily whole body rubbings. (Oil Protein Diet by Lothar Hirneise)

Ingredients
- Enema pot
- Watch
- A bowl to collect oil when you are getting rid of bubbles.
- Towel and tissue
- RO filtered water
- ELDI oil or Flax oil
- Towel or Drip Stand

Procedure

Prepare a place near the toilet, so that if you can't hold the enema, you will be making a quick dash and the shorter distance is better.

Cleansing Enema with Plain water

First of all you should take a plain water enema. Purpose of this enema is cleaning of intestines. It is not a retention enema and is evacuated immediately. For this you may use 500-1000ml (2-4 cups) RO filtered water. As soon as the whole water is inside the rectum, go and sit on the commode and release the water slowly.

Take the oil enema immediately after the water enema

- Use advised (above) amount of ELDI or Flax oil. The oil should be at body temperature. The best test is to dip your little finger into the oil.
- Fill the oil into the enema pot. It takes at least 5 minutes for the bubbles to get out of the tube.
- The enema pot should be hanged on a drip stand about 2-3 feet above your body.
- You need to lubricate the nozzle and anus with Flax oil. When all is ready, lie on your right side in the fetal position. Insert the nozzle into the rectum slowly and carefully with your left hand, and un-pinch the tube.
- If you feel little uncomfortable when the oil is going in, pinch the tube, wait till the feeling passes away, then continue again.
- The oil is much more viscous and moves more slowly. You might need to hold the pot a bit higher to get it to run a bit quicker.
- Once the oil is in, wait and hold it for about 12 minutes. After that slowly turn yourself to left side and hold oil for another 12 minutes. You may listen to music while taking enema.
- When done, it is best to sit on the commode for about 15 minutes with something to read (Skelton).

Coffee Enema

Dr. Max Gerson introduced coffee enema back in the 1930s. In this enema about 500ml of coffee is pushed into rectum, this amount only reaches up to sigmoid colon. There is no loss of minerals and electrolytes in Coffee Enema because their absorption occurs well before sigmoid colon. Coffee enema is even safe for those who are allergic to coffee because it is not absorbed into the systemic circulation. You may take this enema once or twice. It has the following benefits:

- **Powerful and Natural Pain Reliever**
- **Cleansing** - Coffee also acts as an astringent in the large intestine, helps cleanse the colon walls.
- **Toxin Elimination** - The major benefit of the coffee enema is elimination of toxins through the liver. Caffeine, theophylline and theobromine dilate the blood vessels and bile ducts, stimulate the liver to discharge more bile and boost the detoxifying process into high gear and heal inflammation. Indeed, endoscopic studies confirm they increase bile output.
- **Stimulates Liver** - Kahweol and cafestol palmitate found in coffee promote the activity of a key enzyme system called glutathione S-Transferase. This is an important mechanism in the detoxification of carcinogens, as the enzyme group is responsible for neutralizing free radicals. Coffee enema stimulates the activity of this system by 600- 700%.

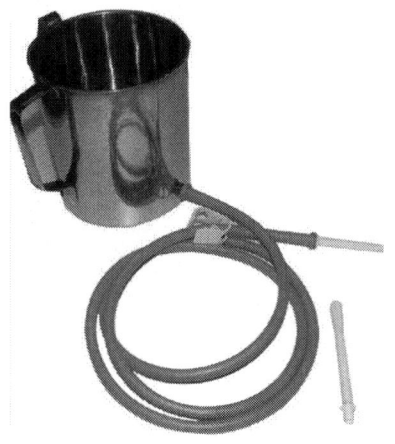

Coffee Enema Procedure
- This enema is retained for 12-14 minutes, during this time blood circulates in liver three times and blood is purified. Coffee enema can be given several times a day, few patients take up to seven times a day. Normally if pain is not relieved it may be taken more than one time. You should relax while taking enema; you may listen to music or read newspaper while relaxing. The best time for coffee enema is either early morning after you passed motion or during the day time.

- Grind organic coffee beans. Put approx. 750ml of filtered water in a steal pan and bring it to boil. Add 2-5 heaped Tbsp coffee powder, 3 Tbsp is ideal. It is roughly 20-25grams. Let it continue to simmer for ten minutes or more and then turn off the burner. Allow it to cool down to a very comfortable, tepid temperature. Test it with your finger. It should be the same temperature as your body's temperature. Filter the coffee with fine mesh steal sieve into a jug. This is approximately 500ml.
- Pour 2 cups (500ml) of coffee into the enema pot. Be sure the plastic hose is clamped tightly. Now open the clamp and grasp, but do not close the clamp on the hose. Place the enema tip in the sink. Hold up the enema bag above the tip until the coffee begins to flow out. As soon as it starts flowing, quickly close the clamp. This expels any air in the tube.
- Lubricate the enema tip with a small amount of coconut oil or KY jelly. Create a comfortable and relaxing atmosphere. After a few days you will thoroughly enjoy this ritual.
- Light a candle, play some light music and most importantly, make sure you are comfortable and warm. We recommend placing a pillow with a washable cover under your head and lying down on a old towel.
- The position preferred is lying on your back. With the clamp closed hang the pot about 3 feet above your belly. We like to hang the enema pot on a drip stand.
- Insert the tip gently into anus and open the clamp slowly. You should relax and breathe. The coffee may take a few seconds to begin flowing. If you develop a cramp, close the hose clamp, turn from side to side and take a few deep breaths. The cramp will usually pass quickly. Usually nothing happens.
- When all the liquid is inside, close the clamp and remove it slowly. Retain the enema for 12- 14 minutes. You may remain lying on the floor.

- After 14 minutes or so, go to the toilet and empty your gut. Take your time. Wash the enema pot and tube thoroughly with soap and water.
- Take more potassium in the form of fruits and vegetable juices if you take coffee enema regularly (S.A.Wilsons.com).

Epsom bath

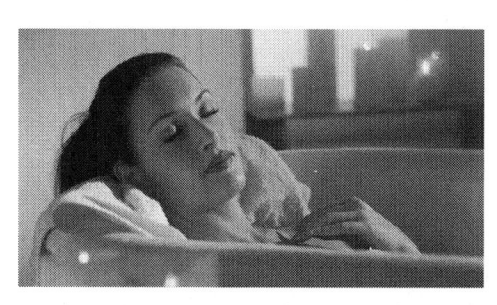

Detoxification of your body through bathing is an ancient remedy that anyone can perform in the comfort of your own home. Your skin is known as the third kidney, and toxins are excreted through sweating. An Epsom salt bath is thought to assist your body in eliminating toxins as well as absorbing the magnesium and nutrients that are in the water. Soaking in Epsom salt actually helps replenish the body's magnesium levels, combating hypertension. The sulfate flushes toxins and helps form proteins in brain tissue and joints. Most of all, it will leave you relaxed, refreshed and awakened. Take it once a week or as advised.

Prepare your bath

- It is a 40 minutes ritual. The first 20 minutes are said to help your body remove the toxins, while the second 20 minutes are for absorbing the minerals from the water
- Fill your tub with comfortably hot water. Use a chlorine filter if possible.
- Add Epsom salt (Magnesium sulfate). For people 50 Kg and up, add 2 cups or more to a standard bath tub.
- Then add 2 cups or more of soda bicarb. It is known for its cleansing ability and even has anti-fungal properties. It also leaves skin very soft.

- Add 2-3 Tbsp ground ginger. While this step is optional, ginger can increase your heat levels, helping to sweat out more toxins. However, since it is heating the body, it may cause your skin to turn slightly red for a few minutes, so be careful with the amount you add. Depending on the capacity of your tub, anywhere from 1 Tbsp to 1/3 cup can be added (Herneise).
- Add aromatherapy oils. Again optional, but there are many oils that will make the bath an even more pleasant and relaxing experience (such as lavender), as well as those that will assist in the detoxification process (tea tree or eucalyptus oil). Around 20 drops is sufficient for a standard bath.
- Swish all of the ingredients around in the tub, and then slip into the tub. You should start sweating within the first few minutes. If you feel too hot, start adding cold water into the tub until you cool off.
- Get out of the tub slowly and carefully. Your body has been working hard and you may get lightheaded or feel weak and drained. On top of that, the salts make your tub slippery, so stand with care.
- Drink plenty of water and relax in bed for a few minutes

Soda bicarb bath

Lothar Hirneise has given lot of importance to Soda bicarb bath. It is thought to assist you in eliminating toxins as well as making your body alkaline so your tumor cells may suffocate. Patient may take it once or even twice a day. Just add 2 cups of soda bicarb in your bath tub filled with warm water and relax in it for 30-40 minutes (Hirneise, 2005).

Sun Therapy

Getting an adequate amount of sunshine is a critical part of Budwig protocol. Once the body has acquired the right oil-protein balance with the Cottage Cheeseand Flax oil, the body develops better capacity to absorb the healing photons from the sun. Remember that for healing of cancer high energy photons from the sun are very important. The sunshine is important to maintain adequate vitamin-D levels in our body. Vitamin-D is a powerful antioxidant that has been linked to preventing many diseases including cancer.

Dr. Budwig's focus was on the importance of photons from the sunbeams and their interaction with vital essential fats (linoleic and linolenic acid) in our body. It is the interaction of photons from the sun and the electrons in proper food that provide the synergistic effect on healing our body. Eating the electron rich Flax oil/Cottage Cheese mixture, must be connected with adequate exposure to sunlight.

There is nothing else on earth with a higher concentration of photons of the sun's energy than man. This concentration of the sun's energy is very much energetic point for humans, with their wave eminently suitable lengths - is improved when we eat electron rich essential oils, which in turn absorbs the photons in the form of electro-magnetic waves of sunbeams.

When you eat the FO/CC mixture, your body becomes a better antenna for the photons from the sunbeam. Your body develops a better ability to absorb the energy from the sun and Transfer it to your cells to perform their vital functions. You become energized at a deep level, and when this happens cancer is healed itself.

It is red light that penetrates deeper in the tissues. In 1968 Dr. Budwig used 695 nm ruby (red) laser light with success to radiate healthy surrounding cancer tissues in cancer patients.

Oil-Protein Diet while travelling

- In her Oil-Protein Diet Cookbook, Dr. Budwig writes: "While traveling, you can always care for yourself with Linomel and hot or cold milk, and/or fruit juices."

- If you are eating a salad in a restaurant, never take the finished dressings, but use olive oil and vinegar. The chance not to take Trans fats is at the least.
- If you want something to be fried, ask the cook to put it in coconut fat or butter. Butter is present in every kitchen.
- Budwig also recommends eating various types of fresh fish to replace the Flax oil and Quark when travelling. You can protect yourself against harm while travelling by ordering fresh fish such as trout, pike, carp and other fresh fish. However, canned (tinned) fish, also shrimps, prawn and other items which frequently contain artificial coloring agents and harmful chemical preservatives, must be strictly avoided.
- Do not eat the "muesli" in hotels. They are mostly denatured carbohydrates.
- Do not use polyunsaturated oils (Flax seed oil, Oil, pumpkin seed oil, etc.) which are kept at room temperature and all contain Trans fatty acids.

For a long vacation

During your long stay travelling away from home, it is really simple to keep up with the Budwig diet, all that is needed was a little bit of preplanning. You may have a fridge and electric tea kettle in the hotel room, or you carry a ice chest.

Wash all fruits and veggies and make enough juice for the travel day and one more day. You should carry a bowl, fork, spoon, sharp knife, and hand blender, nuts, oatmeal and tea. You carry Flax oil, cottage cheese, fruits and veggies in a ice chests for travel.

If you have "eaten something", especially too many carbohydrates in the form of potatoes, rice, noodles or even a "not so healthy dessert/cake", then you should take a walk immediately after eating. (Healing Cancer Naturally)

Making Quark

Quark is a very popular and delicious cheese in Germany. You may find many recipes of making Quark on Google. I am giving you a simple recipe here. In this recipe you will learn how it is easy to make your own homemade Quark.

Ingredients
- 1 liter milk preferably <2% fat
- 500ml cultured buttermilk
- Cheese cloth

Instructions
- In a large glass bowl add milk and buttermilk. Stir well and cover with a clean kitchen towel.
- Let this sit at room temperature for 24 hours. The mixture will thicken slightly.
- Heat the oven to 125^0 F and shut off. Set the bowl uncovered into the oven for about 45 min. The mixture will change to yogurt like texture.
- Add a Cheese cloth to a colander and set on a large bowl.
- Pour the milk mixture into the colander, twist the ends and let drain for about 1 ½ to 2 hours.
- The Quark will be in the towel and the whey will be in the bowl. One liter milk usually yields 200gms of Quark.

Making Cottage Cheese

In some places good quality Cottage Cheese is also not available and you need to make your own. Today I am giving you a very good recipe for home made cottage cheese.

Ingredients
- 1 liter natural, low-fat cow's milk preferably <2% fat
- 1/3 cup Vinegar
- Cold water

Instructions

- Mix 1/3 cup of vinegar in 2 cups of water and keep aside. Diluted vinegar yields soft cheese. You may also use diluted lemon juice.
- Boil the milk in a heavy bottomed pan over medium heat, stirring frequently making sure milk does not burn on the bottom of the pan. As the milk comes to a boil, remove the pan from the gas burner and place it on kitchen counter.
- Now add about a glass of cold water to bring the milk's temperature down to about 75-80 degrees Celsius. We want to curdle the milk at this temperature, so we get a soft cheese.
- Then add little (about 1-2 Tbsp) diluted vinegar slowly and stir the milk gently. After 10 seconds, add little vinegar slowly and stir the milk. Go on adding vinegar until the curd will start separating from the whey. Remember you should curdle the milk slowly.
- Once the cheese has completely separated from the whey, add a glass of cold water and drain the whey using a stainless steel strainer.
- Now Transfer the curdled cheese into a suitable container and blend thoroughly with electric hand blender until you get very smooth and thick creamy cheese. If the cheese is dry, add a little milk while blending. This is your home made cottage cheese.

Buckwheat

Dr. Budwig highly recommended buckwheat in her healing diet. Contrary to its name, this seed is not related to wheat. Buckwheat is a gluten free power food!

Buckwheat is supercharged with health-boosting nutrients and phytochemicals, including B-vitamins, magnesium, manganese, phosphorus, zinc, copper, potassium, and selenium. It is also one of the best natural sources of rutin and D-chiro-

Inositol, two phytochemicals that have been associated with a number of interesting health benefits. It is the best source of high-quality, easily digestible proteins. This makes it an excellent meat substitute. What's more, buckwheat grouts (the hulled kernels) are generally well tolerated and rarely cause allergic reactions or other adverse effects in humans. These gluten-free kernels can be served as an alternative to rice or made into delicious buckwheat porridge.

Studies have shown that populations eating diets high in fiber-rich whole grains and seeds, like buckwheat, consistently have lower risk for colon cancer. Research reported at the American Institute for Cancer Research (AICR) International Conference on Food, Nutrition and Cancer, by Rui Hai Liu, M.D., Ph.D., and his colleagues at Cornell University shows that buckwheat, contain many powerful phytonutrients that can fight cancer.

Energy Healing

Mild exercise

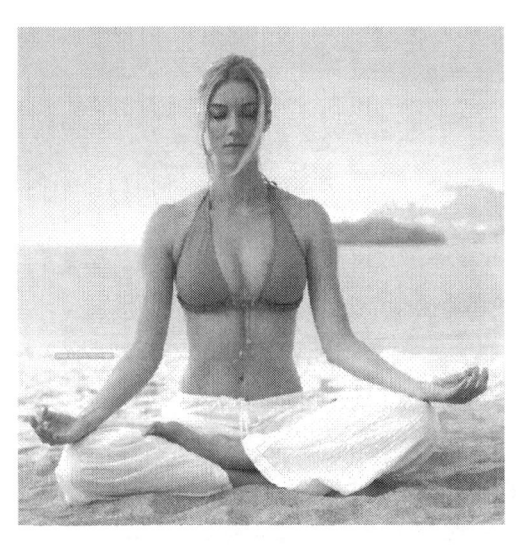

Patient can do mild exercise and remain active if his condition permits. He can go for a walk or do light yoga in the open terrace or garden under the healing and refreshing sunshine. Patient can jog for a few minutes after lunch or dinner. It is very beneficial for cancer patient. But if patient is serious and has metastasis, he should not jog, better he should relax in his house.

Patient can keep himself busy in many activities like sitting in garden enjoying nature, visualization, listening music, reading, laughing, chatting with friends etc. Stress, depression, anxiety, anger and fear can be very damaging to him. Share your feelings with your life partner or a best friend.

You should try your best to remove stress and negative thoughts and balance the flow of energy "prana" or "chi" in your body. Do meditation, Emotional Freedom Technique EFT, Qigong, Reiki, Acupuncture, Acupressure, Sun Salutation etc. to heal your body, mind and spirit.

Meditation

Meditation is a means of Transforming the mind. Meditation practices are techniques that encourage and develop concentration, clarity, positivity, and relaxation of the body and mind. Do any simple meditation for relaxation. Meditation stimulates pineal gland (*piyush granthi*) to shower melatonin hormone. Melatonin controls circadian rhythm and induces restorative sleep. Its powerful antioxidant effect offers important enhancements to the brain and nervous system, helping protect against age-related damage. Melatonin is power anti-stress and anticancer hormone.

Yoga Nidra

It is divine sleep with alertness. In 15 minute yoga nidra session, you relax in a fully supported shavasan, limbs limp, breath quiet, thoughts drifting by. In the distance, the teacher's voice blends with the sound of Tibetan bells. All traces of the day fade away, time stops, and stillness washes over the body. Yoga nidra is a systematic method of complete relaxation, holistically addressing our physiological, neurological, and subconscious needs.

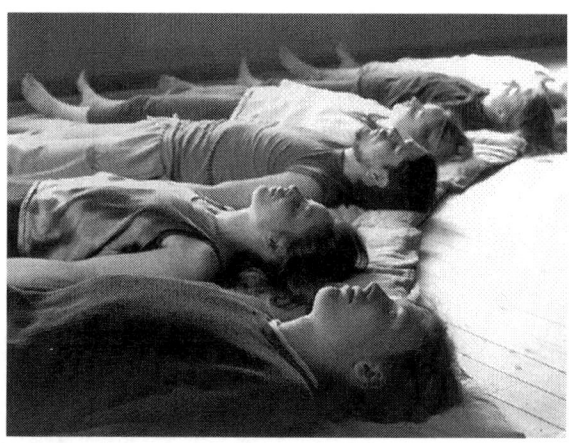

How long should you take this protocol?

If all is well patient feels better and tumor start to shrink within a 3 or 4 months, if he follows treatment religiously and honestly. He may be cured in one or two years. **It is recommended that the Budwig protocol and full diet is followed for at least five years.** Even after that he should maintain healthy eating and life style.

Dr. Budwig has clearly mentioned that if you do not get the desired success, do not blame the protocol, rather try to find out your mistakes and correct them. The threshold between winning and losing is very small, and even a minor mistake can unbalance the complete healing process.

How do I recognize a good Flax seed oil?

Good Flax seed oil is unfortunately dependent on many factors. The IOPDF assigns a star for each fulfilled criterion. The best oil has thus 6 stars and the worst gets no star. Let us look at the 6 criteria in detail:

Criterion 1: Cooling chain

Studies have shown that, in addition to processing the Flax seed, cooling is the most important criterion for a good Flax seed oil. So buy only Flax seed oil stored in a refrigerated rack and kept in a permanent cold chain. If you shop through the Internet, the Flax seed oil must be delivered in a Styrofoam packaging and as fast as possible.

Criterion 2: Local Flax seed

Weekly shipping on ships and sometimes additional chemicals used can cause great damage to Flax seed. Therefore, make sure that you only buy Flax seed oil whose Flax seed comes from the country where you are living or at least from the same continent. This normally can be seen at the seal.

Criterion 3: Omega-3 fatty acid content

The Oil-Protein Diet is about linolenic acid (omega-3). Buy Flax seed oil with a high amount of linolenic acid. Depending in which country you are living the range can be between 55% - 63%.

Criterion 4: Organic quality

It makes a big difference whether Flax seed grows in biologically controlled soil or in soils of conventional agriculture. So buy only Flax seed oils with organic quality, unless you know the oil mill personally and know what Flax seed the mill is processing.

Criterion 5: glass bottle

Flax seed oil and electron differentiation oils are available in glass and plastic bottles or in canisters, which are mostly made of tinplate. Consumers should only buy oils in glass bottles. Avoid plastic bottles, as they may contain highly toxic softeners.

Criterion 6: Light

Flax seed oil should be packaged and stored in a light-proof package. Therefore, only buy bottles in dark brown or dark green bottles. (Oil Protein Diet by Lothar Hieneise)

Linomel

Linomel is an invention by Dr Budwig. Freshly crushed Flax seed is mixed with honey and milk powder so that the crushed Flax seed is more stable. There is no doubt that freshly crushed Flax seed is more valuable, but also has the disadvantage that you do it yourself and clean the grinder afterwards. That is why Linomel still has an existence right. Do not buy crushed Flax seed in the shop as the chance that these contain Trans fatty acids is 100%.

Is there an alternative to Linomel?

- Freshly crushed Flax seed is an alternative. This must be eaten immediately after the meal, otherwise it will oxidize.
- Make your own Linomel. Mix 6 tablespoons freshly crushed Flax seed with a tablespoon of honey. Small tip: Grind the Flax seed, e.g. in a coffee grinder, and set the grinder to coarse. So it mixes better with the honey.

(Oil Protein Diet by Lothar Hieneise)

Questions and Answers

How do I store Flax seed oil?

Generally cool. Best at 5^0-10^0 (Fahrenheit 41-50) in the refrigerator. Always keep the Flax seed oil bottles upright and never lay them down as they may cause faster oxidation.

Should I now buy low fat Quark or Quark with 20% or 40% fat?

Only a Quark with as little fat (less than 2%) is optimal. Quark is about sulfur-containing amino acids. Less fat means more amino acids.

Can Quark be replaced with tofu, yoghurt or soya?

Absolutely no.

Is there an alternative to Quark?

In many books or on the Internet, it is always claimed that there are alternatives to Quark, such as e.g., yogurt, soy or whey protein (which you should never use!). This is wrong. There is absolutely no good substitute for Quark. The only alternative (although it has a slightly different composition like Quark) is Cottage Cheese with as little fat as possible. This should only be used if no Quark is available.

Can I eat cheese?

Basically yes, but in moderation and with the exception of cream cheese and fresh cheese. Only raw milk/hard cheese is permitted. Cheese of sheep or goat is preferable.

Can I eat raisins and dates?

Yes, raisins and dates are allowed in small quantities.

Which fat can be used for frying?

Only coconut fat.

Can I use olive oil?

Theoretically, you can use any organic oils with salad. Dr Budwig preferred Flax seed oil, pumpkin seed oil, wheat germ oil, poppy oil, and thistle oil are also permitted, but do not heat. Oleolox may be heated for two minutes.

Can I drink coffee?

No.

Can soya and oatmeal be eaten?

Dr Budwig wrote several times that oat flakes, soy flakes, yeast flakes and other flakes are permitted. But today I just say that you buy only high quality organic "flakes".

Can I eat bread?

Dr Budwig has recommended her patients to eat no bread during acute tumor phases. Instead, she recommended full-grain rice waffles or Ezekiel bread as an alternative.

Can cows or soy milk be drunk?

No, drinking any milk is forbidden in the Oil-Protein Diet.

Can noodles be eaten?

In the literature of Dr Budwig nearly always did not allow cancer patients to eat noodles. The reason is that noodles are made of flour, eggs and oil. Flour has the disadvantage that it is basically a fast-digesting sugar and mostly the producers use cheap oils. Energetically speaking, noodles are "not really full with electrons". Unfortunately, you are worsening the already bad adrenaline - insulin ratio of a cancer patient.

Which milk can be used for the Quark?

Dr Budwig recommended raw milk. Unfortunately these are nowadays difficult to buy anywhere. Alternatively, pasteurized milk is also okay. All other varieties of milk, such as ultra-heat-treated or homogenized (long life or full cream), are prohibited.

Budwig Diet & Protocol - In Brief

This is raw organic diet with lot of Flax oil and Juices. Consume only clean or RO filtered water. To get the best results, proper guidance is strongly recommended. Below are brief guidelines of the Budwig Diet you don't have to consume all the foods on this list. This information is from Dr. Budwig's books.

First thing in the morning – One glass of sauerkraut juice, preferably raw & homemade. Raw unheated kraut has enzymes, probiotics and vitamins which help the digestive system, metabolize foods & improve immunity.

Just before breakfast - green or herbal tea

Breakfast – First blend 3 Tbsp. Flax oil, 3 Tbsp. milk and a Tsp real honey; then gradually add 6 Tbsp. Quark or Cottage Cheeseand blend. Garnish in layers. Add 2 Tbsp freshly ground Flax seeds n a bowl, then add a layer of crushed fresh fruits, then pour oil cheese mixture and put raw nuts on top. Afterward, if hungry, choose whole grain organic bread, raw vegetables, & quality cheeses such as Edam, Gouda, Emmentaler, Sbrinz or Camembert.

Mid-morning - Homemade vegetable juice (carrots, beets w/lemon or apple, or greens). Homemade carrot or beet juices are very important cancer-fighters.

Before Lunch (especially serious patients) - Champagne with 1 Tbsp ground Flax seeds in small glass of fruit juice. The champagne helps with absorption of the seeds.

Lunch - Salad plate (tomato, cucumber, lettuce, radish, cabbage, broccoli, and pepper) with homemade Cottage Cheeseand Flax oil mayo dressing (prepared by mixing together 2 Tbsp Flax oil, 2 Tbsp milk, 2 Tbsp Cottage Cheeseand 1 Tbsp lemon juice, add a variety of herbs making the plate most appealing.

Lunch - Main Course Vegetables cooked in water, then flavored with oleolox and herbs possibly with oatmeal, curry etc. Vegetable soups flavored with a little oleolox and nutritional yeast flakes, as side dish for buckwheat, brown rice, millet or potatoes.

Lunch Dessert - Must have 2nd serving of 3 Tbsp. Flax oil and 6 Tbsp. Quark or Cottage Cheese with a little milk and honey, well blended. Add raw fruit, fruit juice, raw nuts, and other flavors you like.

Mid-afternoon - 1 Tbsp. freshly ground Flax seed added to 1 glass of pure fruit juice, homemade.

Late afternoon - Papaya or pineapple juice, 1 glass, with 1 Tbsp Flax seeds freshly ground.

Dinner - Grains alone or grains & beans with vegetables with oleolox, nutritional yeast flakes & spices. Eat buckwheat at least 4 days in a week. Grains & beans combined make a complete protein. Vegetables such as spinach, asparagus, broccoli, & cabbage add nutrition and aid absorption. Dine early.

Late Evening - 1 glass red wine (optional). Go to sleep early - before 10 P.M. if possible.

Prohibitions of Budwig Protocol
- No Sugar, no meat, no eggs, no Butter
- No hydrogenated fat and refined oil
- No soya, corn, peanuts and refined table salt
- No frying, no sautéing, no deep frying
- No preservatives and processed Food
- No microwave, Teflon coated and aluminum cookware
- No cosmetics, chemicals and pesticides
- No foam mattress and pillow.
- No nylon, polyester or acrylic clothing, only cotton, silk and wool is allowed.
- No Crt. TV and mobile phones
- No leftover food

Elimination or Detoxification
May include (Remember the Mnemonic - M.Sc. Botany)
- **Flax oil massage,**
- **sun therapy,**
- **coffee enema** and
- **soda bicarb bath,** epsom bath, oil pulling, steam bath, sauna bath, liver, colon and kidney cleansing etc.

Energy Therapies (Remember MTV)
- **Meditation**, Meditation, yoga nidra, positive attitude, system change and deep breathing exercises.
- **Tumor contract** – Tell your tumor that if it grows in size, then you may die, and eventually he also will die. So advise him to become microscopic in size. In return you promise to make some changes in your life so that both of you might live long. If he agrees with your proposal, sign a contract with him immediately.
- **Visualization** – is the most important tool to tap into the power of your imagination to help heal cancer. Remain tuned to your healthy and happy future.

Important and must do therapies with Budwig
- Dandelion root 1 Tsp once or twice a day
- Black seed oil as advised by Maria Hurairah
- Bitter apricot kernels 5 kernels per 5kg of body weight with a Tsp pumpkin seeds
- Essiac tea 30ml to 90ml per day
- Brazil nuts a nut a day
- Nano curcumin 1 cap twice or thrice a day
- and Coenzyme Q-10 1 cap once or twice a day
- Nutritional yeast flakes

Lothar Hirneise

Great supporter of Budwig Protocol

Eleven years, Lothar Hirneise worked as a trained nurse in the State Psychiatric Hospital in Winnenden. After four years, he took psychoanalysis training. Hirneise was also master in Eastern combat sports and a Kung Fu teacher. He owned a successful sporting goods company, which he sold for a tidy profit in 1986. After a year one of his close friend developed Testicular Cancer. Lothar went in search of information about cancer therapies and came across Lynne McTaggart, the founder of the book and magazine "What Doctor's Don't Tell You." Then he was informed that Frank Wiewel, president of the American organization "People Against Cancer", which operates alternative cancer research since 1985, would come to London. So he went to London with his best friend Klaus Pertl to attend this conference for alternative cancer treatments (early 1997). This weekend his friend died. This was the starting point of his intensive quest for potential cancer therapies. He had time and money and read everything he could get his hands on. He nearly went crazy and was severely infected by a virus called Holistic Oncology. He travelled to Bahamas, Mexico, Russia, China, and the United States and all over Europe.

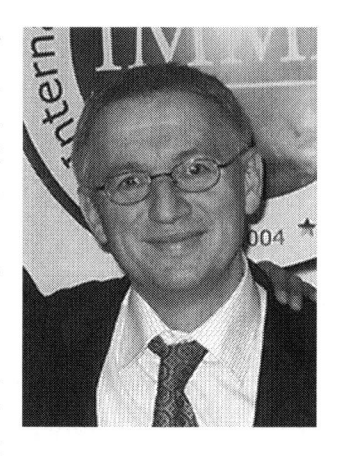

Frank Wiewel advised him to visit Dr. Budwig who lived only 60 km from his home in Germany. Lothar and Klaus Pertl visited Budwig in the spring of 1998, and from the beginning it was an intense relationship that persisted for a very long time.

Over several years he remained in close contact with this great sage of Science. The content of their conversations used to be about fats and electrons. One day she suggested writing a book in which, she could explain her theories again, briefly and concisely. And the Book Cancer - "The Problem And The Solution" was written. Lothar worked very hard in the creation of this great book.

Lothar Hirneise is founder and President of "People Against Cancer", Germany. He is a great researcher and writer on alternative healing. In his book "Chemotherapy cures cancer and the earth is flat" he puts an "Encyclopedia of unconventional cancer treatments", and summarizes the results of his years of worldwide research together. The book became a best seller within no time. He had successfully treated thousands of cancer patients at his center in Germany (3E Zentrum, Buocher Höhe Im Salenhäule 10, D-73630 Remshalden-Buoch Telefon: 07151-98130).

Tumor is not a problem, but a solution

Lothar Hirneise says: "A tumor is the body's solution to some problem in your body. A tumor forms because someone is no longer producing adrenaline, which is needed to break down sugar. An excess of sugar is dangerous, so the body produces tumors. Tumors ferment or burn sugar. Tumors also use a lot of energy - sugar - due to the fast division of cells. Cancer cells function like liver cells, but much more efficiently. So the tumor helps you to get rid of poisons from your body. Without the tumor you would be really ill. That is why you shouldn't immediately operate to remove a tumor. First strengthen and detoxify yourself. If the tumor still continues to grow - which is almost never the case - you can always operate later."

3E Program

He travels a lot in search of finding most successful alternative cancer therapies. In the last few years he has interviewed several hundred final stage so-called survivors, meaning patients who were in the final stage of cancer and who are all healthy again today. Based on his findings he proposed a 3E Program for cancer.

- Eat well
- Eliminate the toxins from the body
- Energy

He noticed that 100% of all survivors, did the energy work. In approximately - say 80% of all patients, He found a change in diet. And in at least 60% of all patients, took intensive detoxification rituals. This is the basis of his, so much talked about 3E Program for healing cancer.

Diet and Nutrition

He proudly says that he has shaken the hands with hundreds of people, who made extreme dietary change and became well. They are still alive and living a healthy life. If you still believe that Cancer diets are nonsense, go to him, he will prove the opposite. He has interviewed enough patients and knows them personally. Good nutrition naturally means getting energy. He explains that we have three ways and means of getting energy into our bodies.

1. The first is the light. Light is naturally our number one source of energy. He is 100% sure.

2. The second way is organic nutrition. He emphasized strict organic diet; of course, you do not get any energy from a chicken burger. Rather, when you eat this, you lose some energy, which you have to compensate later.

3. Another possibility which you have is let the energy flow in your body, in your meridians and in your thoughts. Think

about the feeling you had last time when you were in love. You felt wonderful; you were on top of the sky. But what did it change? Did your DNA change? Did your cell respiration change? Nothing really changed. The Indians would say your chakras were opened and the energy started to flow freely again. This is the secret, not only to get the energy, but also to let it flow freely. This proves that our thoughts, our mental-spiritual side is too important.

Now back to nutrition. Out of all nutritional therapies of cancer that he had investigated, the Budwig diet is definitely number one. He investigated thousands of patients, Dr. Budwig allowed him to investigate all her cases of the last thirty years, and he concluded that nowhere you find such fantastic cases as with Dr. Budwig, not even remotely. It's amazing. Even patients who were in coma, when received her Oil-Protein Diet, and rubbed so-called electron differential oils (ELDI oils) on the body, did again come out from coma. They were able to eat, walk and live normally today. It is really miraculous. Therefore, her Oil-Protein Diet became the basis of his 3-E Program for cancer patients.

Detoxification

Next important point that he suggests is detoxification. Detoxification actually covers two points.

1. The first is naturally to avoid toxins and poisons e.g. use of cosmetics, toothpaste, etc.

2. And the second point which belongs to detoxification is not to add any toxins in future. The most important point is definitely diet. It doesn't need further explanation. We are ingesting lot of poisons through our diet. Is better not to eat than all this rubbish that one can buy today.

Healthy teeth and gums are phenomenally important. Heat is a very good way to expel poisons. All the parasite cleanses, colon cleansing, ELDI oils, drinking a lot of water is essential. Going out into the sun light, twice daily is very important. You might have listened today that the sun is suddenly bad for you and may cause skin cancer. That is nonsense, forget it. We are all children of the light, we definitely need the light. Even if it's raining and cloudy today go outside. Even if patient is in coma, he must be wheeled out. You should go twice daily into the light. Light increases Vitamin D levels, important for the liver and increases energy levels.

Energy Work

Energy work is the most important point. He divides it into mental and spiritual work. Naturally, you are advised to do meditation and develop positive thinking. You think about life, 'Why do I have cancer and what is the purpose of my life, why am I here on this earth?' and so on. But he focused on something what he called the **SYSTEM CHANGE**. He explains that we all live in Systems. In our marriage, in our house, in our job, etc. Many, many, many of these cancer patients made system jumps. Means that they kicked their husband in the butt and threw him out. They quit their job, they moved, they not only moved their bed, they moved out of their apartment, went to other countries. Quite honestly, I don't know, what should you do? But Lother's experience is that it it's remarkable to what extent people changed their life before they were in a position to get well.

Lothar Hirneise Concludes: "There is no spontaneous remission, there are only people who positively change their life and regained their health that way." (Hirneise, 2005)

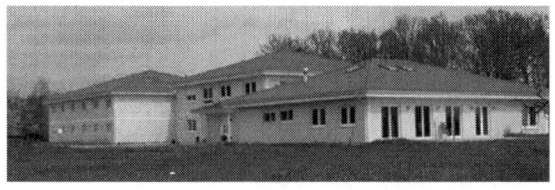

~~**~~

Interview of Dr. Johanna Budwig

Lothar Hirneise worked with Dr. Johanna Budwig from 1998 to 2003. He explained that there is much more available to cancer patients than just chemo and irradiation. Mr. Lothar Hirneise conducted this great interview in 1998 (Budwig, Cancer The Problem And The Solution).

Lothar Hirneise: What is your fundamental research?

Dr Johanna Budwig: In 1949, I developed Paper Chromatography of fats with Professor Kaufmann, the director of the Federal Institute for Research on Grain, Potatoes and Fat, and my former doctoral advisor, who was also director of the Pharmaceutical Institute. With this technique for first time I was able to detect fats, fatty acids and lipoproteins directly even in 0.1 ml of blood. I used Co 60 isotopes successfully to produce the first differential reaction for fatty acids, and produced the first direct iodine value via radioiodine. I also developed control of atmosphere in closed system by using gas systems which act as antioxidants. I further developed Coloring, separating effects of fats and fatty acids. I too studied their behavior in blue light, red light with fluorescent dyes.

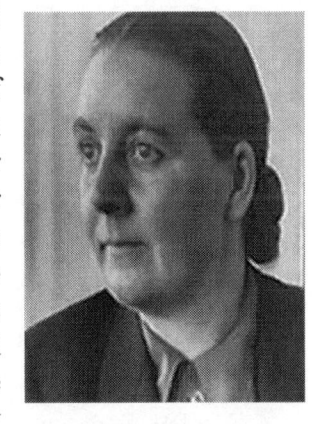

Using rhodamine red dye, I studied the electrical behavior of the unsaturated fatty acids with their "halo". With this technique I could prove that electron rich highly unsaturated Linoleic and Linolenic fatty acids (Flax oil being richest source) were the mysterious and undiscovered decisive fats in respiratory enzyme function which Otto Warburg could not find. I studied the electromagnetic function of pi-electrons of the linolenic acid in the cell membranes, for all nerve function, secretions, mitosis, as well as cell division. I also examined the synergism of the sulfur containing protein with the Pi-electrons of the highly unsaturated fatty acids and their significance for the formation of the hydrogen bridge between fat and protein, which represent "the only path" for fast and focused Transport of electrons during respiration.

This immediately caused an excitement in scientific community. Everybody thought that it will open new doors in Cancer research. I also proved that Hydrogenated fats, refined oils including all Trans fatty acids were not having any vital electrons and thus proved as respiratory poisons. We published this research exclusively in many journals including "New Directions in Fat Research".

Lothar Hirneise: What is the prime cause of Cancer?

Dr Johanna Budwig: In 1928 Dr. Otto Warburg proved that all normal cells require oxygen absolutely, but cancer cells can live without oxygen. It is a rule without exception. If you deprive a cell 35% of its oxygen for 48 hours and it would become cancerous. Dr. Otto Warburg has proved it clearly that the root cause of cancer is lack of oxygen in the cells, which creates an acidic state in the human body.

He also discovered that cancer cells are anaerobic i.e. do not breathe oxygen, get the energy by fermentation of glucose producing lactic acid and cannot thrive in the presence of high levels of oxygen. Long back in 1911 Swedish scientist Torsten Thunberg postulated that sulfur containing protein (found in cottage cheese) and some unknown fat is required to attract oxygen in the cell. This fat plays a major role in the cellular respiration. For nearly half century scientists were trying to identify this unknown and mysterious fat but nobody succeeded.

Lothar Hirneise: How did you develop cancer therapy which is called Budwig Protocol?

Dr Johanna Budwig: During my research I found that the blood of seriously ill cancer patients had deficiency of unsaturated essential fats (Linoleic and Linolenic fatty acids), lipoproteins, phosphatides, and hemoglobin. I also noticed that cancer patients had a strange greenish-yellow substance in their blood which is not present in the blood of healthy people. I wanted to develop a healing program for cancer.

So I decided to straight way go for human trials and I enrolled 642 cancer patients from four big hospitals in Münster. I started to give Flax oil and Cottage Cheeseto the cancer patients. After just three months, patients began to improve in health and strength, the yellow green substance in their blood began to disappear, tumors gradually receded and at the same time as the nutrients began to rise. Thus I had a cure for cancer. It was a great victory and the first milestone in the battle against cancer. My treatment is based on the consumption of Flax seed oil with low fat cottage cheese, raw organic diet, detoxification, mild exercise, Flax oil massage and the healing powers of the sun. I have treated approx. 2500 cancer patients during last few decades. Prof. Halme of surgery clinic in Helsinki used to keep records of my patients. According to him my success was over 90% and this too was achieved in cases where conventional Oncology failed.

Lothar Hirneise: Can you tell us more about the unsaturated fatty acids and their net-like connections?

Dr. Johanna Budwig: Fatty acid is a carboxylic acid having unbranched chain of 4 to 28 carbons. The saturated fatty acids have primarily short carbon chains. In butter, coconut fat, goat fat and sheep fat the fatty acids consists of 4, 6, 8, 10 or 12 carbons. These fats are saturated, however they can also easily metabolize if the essential fatty acids are present. The unsaturated vital fatty acids really start with the chain with 18 carbon compounds. There are also fatty acids with up to 30 carbons. Fatty acids with 18 carbons, like in Flax oil with the higher level of unsaturation, are more important for human beings, particularly for the brain functions of man. Linoleic acid rich in electrons is considered vital. There is particularly high amount of energy in this double double bonds of the linoleic acid.

This energy wanders and is not fixed in place while in a chemical compound, such as with table salt the energy is fixed. This energy, wandering between electrons and the positively charged protein with sulfur groups is an alternating association process in the electromagnetic field. This is very important. Perhaps you are familiar with the painting of Michelangelo, where God creates Adam (two fingers pointing to each other, however they do not touch). This is quantum physics, here the fingers do not touch. The physicists who I know, Max Planck, or Albert Einstein, or Dessauer all represent the view that man is created by God in His image. You see in being together as human beings there is certainly also a connection without directly touching the other person. The dipolarity with a single double bond in olive oil is weaker than it is in sunflower seed oil, which is has two double bonds. This double double bond is considered to be vital for man. However if the same chain length of 18 carbons has three unsaturated fatty acid double bonds, then the electrical energy is as strong as a magnet. This electronic energy is negatively charged. The positively charged sulfur groups of the protein adhere in the unsaturated bonds where the electrons are and that is where they insert their sulfur-containing compounds.

This produces the lipoproteins. The life process is sustained in the interplay between the positively-charged particles and negatively-charged particles. In this process there is no connection, and this is our life element. If radical damage occurs at this point through fatty acids that has lost electron energy, but rather are cross-linked like a net, then the dipolarity can no longer work actively in this net. This is the deadly effect of free radicals, because instead of the chains with the electron clouds they interlace like a net without electron clouds, indeed with unsaturated bonds, but without dipolarity. I quickly knew that the triple unsaturated fatty acids, which were called linolenic acid, and which no one had isolated before me, had 18 carbons and that they did not always carry their double bonds at the same point. They have such a strong electronic energy compared to the heavier matter in the 18-link fatty acid chains, that biologically this energy is far greater than it is with the next arachidonic acid with 20 links. The highest electron collection is with the combination of linoleic-linolenic fatty acids in Flax oil. The linolenic acid as conjugated (interaction of neighboring double bonds in the molecule that are separated by a single bond) fatty acid is even more effective and is even more strongly interplay with linoleic acid as it is present in the Flax oil for oxygen absorption. This was relatively easy for me to verify in my experiments. I would like to emphasize this. The combination of double unsaturated linoleic acid with triple unsaturated linolenic acid is particularly well-combined in Flax seed.

Lothar Hirneise: Is it this energy that heals cancer?

Dr. Johanna Budwig: Yes, this energy is now movable and it is easily released. It is precisely this energy that heals cancer, or does not even allow it to occur. If this vital element is present then no tumor can exist. This vital element is a deciding factor in the immune system. There is no effective factor in the immune system other than the essential fatty acids.

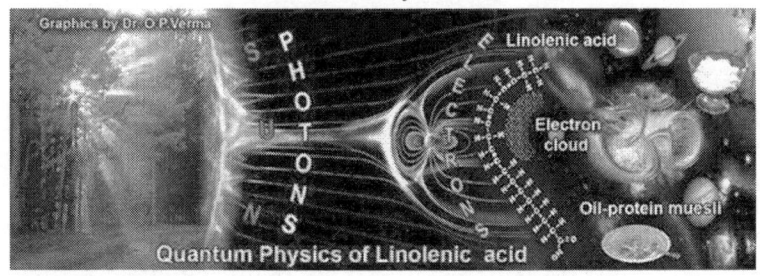

Lothar Hirneise: What is an electron cloud?

Dr Johanna Budwig: If the enhancement of electronic energy is always higher through absorption of sun photons in the unsaturated fatty acids e.g. in linolenic fatty acids, then the power of the electrons is so high in the dipolarity between gravity and electrons, that they lifts off of the heavy mass and floats like a cloud hence I called them electron cloud.

Lothar Hirneise: What is the significance of the cloud?

Dr. Johanna Budwig: No life form has as much energy to store the electrons and photons as doe's man. The electronic energy stored particularly in the vital, highly unsaturated fatty acids, is very strong life element for man. Man cannot live without them. If oils are treated with heat and harsh chemicals (during refining and hydrogenation process to increase their shelf life) then the wealth of vital electronic energy is destroyed and Trans fats are formed with net like connections. They are no longer vital fats with 18 carbons, but rather they form cross-links between the fatty acids like a large net, and are highly damaging to our body, do not adhere with proteins, do not attract oxygen and act like a free radicals. I repeat because it is so important: I have detected particles in oils treated with steam, which indeed have a positive iodine value, but which are highly toxic for man.

Lothar Hirneise: So you preach against these toxic hydrogenated and refined oils?

```
      H  H           H  H             H
      |  |           |  |             |
    -C--C-         -C==C-          -C==C-
      |  |                             |
      H  H                             H

  Saturated Fat   Unsaturated Fat    Trans fat
```

Dr. Johanna Budwig: I am completely against using these "pseudo" fats - "hydrogenated" or "partially hydrogenated". These are the biggest enemy of mankind. I had scientific proofs. The heart rejects these fats and they are deposited as inorganic fat on the heart muscle itself. They end up blocking circulation, damage heart action, inhibit cell renewal and impede the free flow of blood and lymph fluids.

But it was highly profitable business for multinationals. When I preached against these fats, they stood against me, first they tried to bribe me and when I refused they filed many fake court cases against me. I was working for humanity and had scientific proof. I was like rock of Gibraltar in my decision; I fought and won all the cases ultimately.

Lothar Hirneise: What is your view point about surgery for tumors?

Dr. Johanna Budwig: I am totally against radiation and chemo; I also reject hormonal treatment. Surgery must be considered individually. I am not a proponent of quickly making artificial anus. Conventional oncology no longer does justice to the cancer patients.

Lothar Hirneise: You also studied medicine at the age of 47 years.

Dr. Johanna Budwig: (smiling) Yes handsome! That's right, my opponents were accusing me that how can I treat cancer patients without a doctors degree. This thing pinched me, so in 1955, I joined medical school in Göttingen. There I was using my therapy very successfully in various clinics. I still remember the time I was working late one night in Göttingen, a woman came to me, with her small child whose arm was supposed to be amputated due to a tumor. I treated her and soon the subject of amputation was dismissed and the child quickly did very well.

Because I was still a medical student at this time, I was summoned to appear before the Municipal Court due to a petition that I should be prohibited from studying medicine. I explained the truth in the court. The judge rejected the case and said, "You have done a good job, Budwig. In my area of jurisdiction nothing will happen to you. If it does there will be a scandal in the scientific community."

Lothar Hirneise: What do you recommend for prevention of cancer?

Dr. Johanna Budwig: Consume only Flax oil as oil. I reject frozen and preserved meat. Fresh meat is OK. No frozen food and no bakery products. Avoid all Trans fats. Eat organic diet. Oleolox should be used as butter. Prepare fruit juices yourself. Cheese and potatoes are OK. Also the electromagnetic environment (e.g. microwave and mobile phones etc.) in which we live is very important. I reject synthetic textiles and foam mattresses because they steal lot of electrons from you. A lot of wood in home construction and woolen or silk carpets are also important. Wear gemstones, they also have good biological radiation. Books could be written on gemstones. The environment and living conditions must be as biological (organic & natural) as possible. Regular sleep is very important.

Sun, Photons and Electrons

Sun, photons, electrons - What are they?

Sun rays reach the earth as an inexhaustible source of energy. The sources of power in mineral oil, coal, green plant-foods and fruits are based on the energy supplied by the sun's radiation. Light is the fastest traveler from star to star. There is nothing that travels faster than light. Light speeds along with time. Physicists emphasize that the photon, the quantum, the smallest component of the sun's rays is eternal. It is truly a life element. Life is impossible without the photon.

The photon is always in motion. Nothing can ever halt its motion. The photon is full of colors and can change its color, its frequency, when present in large numbers. The photon - acknowledged to be the purest form of energy, the purest wave, always in motion—can unite with a second photon, when it is in resonance with the other, to form a "short-lived particle." This particle, known as "O" particle, can break up into two photons again, without mass, as a pure wave in motion. This is the basis for the wonderful back and forth movement between light and matter. This photon can never be pinned down to one location. This is the foundation for the Theory of Relativity. The photon gave rise to Max Planck's and Einstein's formation of the quantum theory which is of such significance today.

Electrons

Electrons are a smallest particles of matter and are in continual movements. They vibrate continually on their own wavelength. They have their own frequency, like radio receivers which are set at a certain wavelength. The electron orbits in matter around a nucleus. The heavy matter in the nucleus (proton) is charged with positive electricity. In contrast to this, the electron carries a negative charge. The positively charged nucleus and the negatively charged electron attract each other by means of their electrical opposition. But the electron, always in motion, never approaches the nucleus close enough to be drawn out of its own orbit. It maintains a certain freedom of movement within its prescribed orbit.

The electron loves photons. It attracts photons by its magnetic field. When an electrical charge moves, it always produces a magnetic field. The moving photon also has a magnetic field. Both fields, the magnetic field of the electrons and the magnetic field of the photons attract each other when the wavelengths are in tune. The wave length of the photon—which the photon can change—must fit into the wavelength of the orbiting electron so that the orbit maintains a complete wavelength. This feature is extremely interesting in terms of its physical, biological and even philosophical consequences. Matter always has its own vibration, and so, of course, does the living body. The absorption of energy must correspond to one's own wavelength.

Sunbeams are very much in harmony with human. It is no coincidence that we love the sun. The quantum biologists say that the resonance in our body is so strongly tuned to the sun's energy that: There is nothing else on earth with a higher concentration of photons of the sun's energy than man. This concentration of the sun's energy with their highly suitable wavelengths is improved when we eat electron-rich food. The electrons attract the electromagnetic waves of sunbeams. Flax seed oil contain high amount of electrons which are on the wavelength of the sun's energy. Scientifically, these oils are even known as electron-rich essential highly unsaturated fats. *The famous Quantum Physicist Dessauer writes: If it were possible to increase' the concentration of solar electrons tenfold in this electron-rich unsaturated fats, then man would be able to live 10,000 years.*

The sun's energy and man as an antenna

Almost everyone knows what an antenna is. The marvelous science of Maxwell, the physicist, concerning electro-magnetic waves today are well-researched and of practical use. Famous examples are telegraphy, radio, television, microwave oven, cell phones and various applications of high-frequency technology in the manufacturing of electromagnets, the atom bomb and research into nuclear power as a source of energy. Maxwell was able to show that an electric current flowing in an electrically conductive matter produces a magnetic field. Also electrically conductive matter which is moved within a magnet's field, will produce a current. When an atomic particle, such as an electron, is accelerated by an electric field, this produces electric and magnetic fields, which travel at right angles to each other, produces electromagnetic wave. These fundamental, elementary laws can also be applied to biological processes.

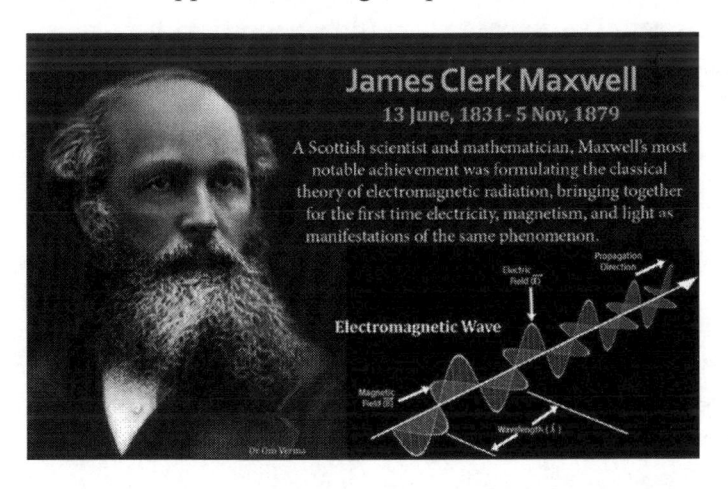

James Clerk Maxwell
13 June, 1831- 5 Nov, 1879

A Scottish scientist and mathematician, Maxwell's most notable achievement was formulating the classical theory of electromagnetic radiation, bringing together for the first time electricity, magnetism, and light as manifestations of the same phenomenon.

When the sun shines on the leafy canopy of a tree and is absorbed through photosynthesis, this causes movement in the electrical charge of the electrons. A magnetic field is also brought about when the water in trees rises. When we, with our wealth of electrons and conductive living substance, move through the electro-magnetic field of a forest, then a charging with solar electrons takes place in us. When our blood circulates, there is a movement of the electrical charge in the magnetic fields (for example, on the surface lipids of red blood corpuscles), which then causes much induction and re-induction of energy.

With each heartbeat, a dose of the body's own electron-rich, highly unsaturated fats from the lymph system, together with lymph fluid, goes into the blood vessels and thereby into the heart. This constantly stimulates and strengthens the electro-motoric functioning of the heart; Even the movement of the bloodstream is connected with radiation of electromagnetic waves-in accordance with the fundamental law of nature which governs electro-magnetic waves. This Transmitter within humans is always in action.

This Transmitter is also observed in neurons. The cylindrical structure of our nerves with the different layers and ganglions, with the difference in electrical potential between the neurons and dendrites, immediately supplies the picture of how strongly an electric current in a magnetic field leads to the emitting of electromagnetic waves. When I think a positive thought about another person, this involves the emitting of electromagnetic waves. The reception of thought also depends on the wavelength to which the receiver is tuned. There are amplifiers, as well as Transmitters that interfere. This encompasses a whole host of situations that are known under different names such as telepathy, hypnosis, mental telepathy, and many others.

Among Nordic peoples, it is known that the isolated native inhabitants use a tree to amplify thought Transmission, for example, to inform the husband who had gone to town, that he should bring back some salt. Bismark described how, during periods of trouble or pressure, he found relaxation by putting his arms around a tree and leaning his forehead against the trunk. In both cases, it involves electromagnetic waves that behave in accord with Maxwell's mathematical equations.

Fats Syndrome

The special relationship between photons, electrons and Essential Fats (EFAs) described by Dr. Budwig is due to the amazing molecular structures of LA (cis-linoleic acid) and ALA (cis-linolenic acid). The cis-configuration allows de-localized electron clouds (pi-electrons) to collect in the bend produced on the chain. The resulting electrostatic force enables the EFAs to capture oxygen molecules and hold proteins within cell membranes. Like static electricity in a capacitor these charges can produce measurable bioelectric currents essential to nerve, muscle, heart and membrane functions. EFAs are extremely important to the body's overall energy exchange potential — the flow of life force.

Let us concentrate on the actual fats syndrome with its effects on the brain and nerve functions, the organs of the senses, the secretion of mucous, the functioning of the stomach and intestinal tract, liver, gall bladder and kidneys, the lymph and blood vessels, the skin, respiration, the immunity system, the fertilization processes and sexuality. All of these systems and processes of the human being are very much connected with electron-rich highly unsaturated fats, as receivers, amplifiers and Transmitters of electro-magnetic waves, and as supervisor of the vital functions. *The famous Quantum Physicist Dessauer writes: If it were possible to increase the concentration of solar electrons tenfold in this electron-rich unsaturated fat molecule, then man would be able to live 10,000 years.*

Anti-Mensch

Physicists interpret from mathematical formulae that man, with his wealth of electrons, is directed forward in time, which conceals within him the greatest potential to attract the sun's energy, and is directed against entropy. By means of these mathematical formulae, applied to Physics, and by reversing time, the mirror image of human beings is coined—the "Anti-Mensch", lacking electrons, lacks power and strength and directed into the past. It increases the occurrence of cancer. His thought processes, too—is paralyzed, because the element of life, the sun-attuned electrons, is missing.

The process by which x-rays, gamma rays, atom bombs or cobalt rays are set in motion is also equally directed toward the development of the "Anti-Mensch". The electronic structure of the vital functions is destroyed by such rays. According to Feynman's "World Line Diagram" and modern theory of relativity, time and space have been given a relationship in a formula. The "Anti-Mensch" is directed into the past. Human's body tissues with its interplay between solar energy photons and large number of electrons, with its concentration of photons in life's activities and in the dynamics of the vital functions, are directed into the future.

But, when people began to hydrogenate the oils to increase their shelf-life; no-one thought about the consequences of this. In this process these vitally important electrons were destroyed. During hydrogenation, vegetable oils are reacted with hydrogen gas at high temperature. A nickel is used to speed up the reaction and unsaturated fats are hardened. This negative aspect concerning the development of the "Anti-Mensch" is in accordance with Feynman's "World Line Diagram". I emphasize that it means the fats and oils which have had their electron structure destroyed serve, within time and space, to promote the development of the "Anti-Mensch".

The electrons as resonance system

The electrons in our food serve as the resonance system for the sun's energy. Their electro-magnetic field attracts the photons in sunlight. The physicist cannot imagine life without these active and vital photons. These photons, which are in resonance with the electrons in seed oils, are focused on the same wavelength as the sun's energy, serve the life element. This interplay of solar energy photons and the electrons in seed oils governs all the vital functions. Fats are the dominant factor for all the vital functions, according to Ivar Bang.

The electrons of highly unsaturated fats from seed oils, which are on the same wavelength as sunlight, are capable of drawing solar energy and storing it, then, upon demand, of activating it as the purest energy in the form of the electrons clouds, and making it available for the vital functions. All the vital functions are closely connected with membrane function.

The exchange of electrons, the distribution of energy in the whole organism is dependent on these membrane functions — in the nerve pathways, the brain, in every organ, the liver, gall bladder and pancreas in the stomach's mucous membrane and in the kidneys and intestinal tract. The controlling functions of these membranes with their electro-motoric power, is felt everywhere. This is also true for the respiratory functions, and in oxygen absorption and utilization. It also applies to cell division — to all normal growth processes. It is true for the catabolism of substance in the elimination processes taking place by way of the kidneys, intestinal tract and also for the growth of hair and nails, as well as for the development of young life in the womb. Most significant point is that it is this electronic energy that heals cancer. This turning point in the field of proven successful cancer therapy is only one aspect of much bigger picture of the Quantum Biology. A lot of mysteries and miracles have yet to be discovered by doing research in Quantum Biology.

How can we once more reach the peak of human development?

Freeing you from the influences and effects of radiation and from environmental factors which promote development into the "Anti-Mensch", seem important. These goals, set by the individual who chooses, or by the state and food industries with their organization and planning, should be to see that the food we eat consists of electron-rich nutrition. An electron-rich food intake which supplies us with the resonance system for the sun's energy, must once more achieve priority. Such food, as the life element, promotes our sun-attuned energy. This in turn promotes our development, in space and time, into the future. The entire self can then grow and continue to develop further until, in accordance with the laws of nature which govern light and life, the highest level of our being is achieved. *(Excerpted from Dr Johanna Budwig's book "Flax Oil as a True Aid Against Arthritis, Heart Infarction, Cancer and Other Diseases.")*

Daylight

Dr Budwig focused upon the importance of daylight to our health. It is not enough to absorb electrons only through food, but it is important that we feed ourselves so that our cells are able to absorb and process the light coming from the sun. The more sickly someone is, the sooner he is "in the house", which can be a catastrophic mistake. Especially when people are already in a very late stage of the illness, they are often not able to eat enough and good advice is then very difficult. In such cases, Dr Budwig advises to concentrate on the following three points:
- ELDI oils as whole body rubbings and if possible as enemas
- Only freshly squeezed juices and distributed as food throughout the day if possible the breakfast muesli in different variants
- Stay outside as much as possible

You will experience me to explain what to do next. I have been able to see in my life how Dr Budwig's theoretical considerations work when put to practice, if indeed, if they are consistently carried out. If you could experience such a case yourself, and how quickly it can be better for a seriously ill person, you can see Dr Budwig's words in a very different light.

But other great researchers had also dealt with the subject of light long before Dr Budwig. For example, the anthroposophist Rudolf Steiner wrote, about 50 years earlier that there is a fundamental being of our material existence of the earth, of which all materiality has come only through condensation. Every matter on earth is condensed light! There is nothing in material existence, which is something else than condensed light in some form. Wherever you go and feel matter, you have condensed light everywhere. Compressed light. Matter is light by its very nature. In as much as a man is a material being, he is woven of light. Rudolf Steiner and Dr Budwig have pointed out in their writings over and over again the importance of light and that we humans are now heliotropes, which need light and use light. But I have nowhere else than with Dr Budwig so clearly and understandably read, WHY this is and above all, how the charging of the life battery works and / or what importance mainly the linolenic acid or electron clouds play. Because it is so important, I would like to repeat here again: The sicklier someone is, the more he should be in the open." (Oil-Protein Diet by Lothar Hirneise)

Visualization - Path to wellness

The visualization is perhaps the most important tool to tap into the power of your imagination to help heal cancer, manage problems or rather achieve anything in your life. Learning to direct and control images in your mind can help you to relax. This may help to

- Relieve stress
- Control some of the symptoms caused by your cancer or cancer treatments
- Boost your immune system to help your body fight off infections and promote healing

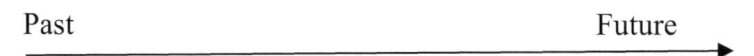

Past   Future
───────────────────────────────→

Whatever you see around yourself is just a vision in the beginning, For example the cup of coffee you are holding in your hands or the house in which you live today did not exist in the past. Not very long ago there was a thought in your mind that you want to construct a dream house for living. Then you made construction designs and all sort of workup. Our whole life runs on the rails of time and never turns back. This is our time line.

First of all understand that everything around us is just a thought, energy or a wave. It is significant to understand this. Then only you will believe that energy can be converted in to a matter. Just imagine that a hypnotist puts a coin on your palm and makes you believe that it is hot. You feel burning in your palm. You may even have blisters on your palm. Here the temperature of coin just changed through only.

If you have believed that certain thought can change the condition of your body within seconds. Then why not a good thought can heal your tumor. In many studies Visualization trainer Carl Simomton has proved that cancer patients live twice if they follow visualization technique systematically.

Lothar Hirneise, the student of Dr. Johanna Budwig, respects Carl's research too much except a few points. Simomton teaches his cancer patients to visualize that their white cells are attacking cancer cells and killing them. Lothar is against this school of thought. Because in this situation patient focuses on his tumor. But Lothar says that main problem is something else, tumor problem is secondary. Secondly patient thinks of a war with a cancer cell, while Lothar believes that cancer patient needs balance and harmony rather than thinking of a war.

Lothar has interviewed hundreds of cancer survivors and came to the conclusion that cancer patient avoids direct confrontation with his tumor, but wants to remain busy in dealing with healthy and happy future. Though every patient has different approach, but end is same, creating a happy future. Lothar admits that visualization is the single most important therapy in his so much talked about 3E Program. After all if we will not create a healthy future for us then who else will do.

Please, review your time line again and compare it with thought-matter line. You will notice that both lines travel in the same direction and never turn back. You can never change the direction of any line. So start now and create your own happy future yourself.

Thought	Matter
──────────────────────────────▶	
Past	Future
──────────────────────────────▶	

I am going to discuss Lothar's technique in detail, which he learned from Europe's famous Visualization trainers Jack Black from Glasgow. Jack has taught his Mind Store System to 50,000 people in last few years. He is consultant of many celebrities and several companies. Lothar recommends that every cancer patient should attend seminars of Jack Black or Klaus Partl. Klaus Partl is right hand of Lothar Hirneise and teaches visualization at his 3E Center in Germany.

Initially Cancer patient thinks that the most important job is to destroy tumor. If he gets rid of tumor then he can plan to take some holistic treatments e.g. visualization. This is very bad decision. It is very important to follow visualization techniques as a part of your tumor destruction program.

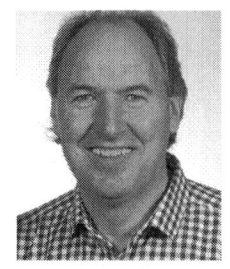

But How does it work? This word HOW is very important, because it usually prevents us to take right decisions. At this moment don't try to think how visualization shall work, how it is going to destroy your tumor. Time being I just say that try to trust us that it actually works.

In short I just say that you learn how to make your future healthy and cheerful, do not focus on present and past. Lothar says that if you know your past, it is easier to change your future. But your main focus should be to create happy future.

Your dream house where you heal your cancer

To give positive impact on your body and mind, it is very important that you become completely relaxed before you start thinking and visualizing. Relaxation or rather achieving alpha stage is the first step. Alpha means relaxed stage (7-14 hertz waves) of your mind. You can relate it with the alpha waves of an EEG tracing. Then there are beta, theta and delta waves. To reach this state there are many techniques or meditations. Some books and CDs are also available. Even listening classical music, meditation or mild yoga can relax you.

When you achieve deep relaxation, start thinking and visualizing. You start it by walking slowly along the right bank of a river. After a short distance you turn towards right. You see blue sky and green meadows. There are lot of trees and a very beautiful house with red terrace. (can imagine your dream house)

Now you enter this house. First room is a beautiful bathroom with a shower. You start taking shower. It washes out all your negativity, toxins and dis-eased cells. After taking shower you sit under the sun, the sunshine dries and fills you with energy within a couple of moments.

Now you go to screen room. On the blank wall of this room there are 3 big LCD monitors. You can relax on the comfortable sofa. You can control these screens with a remote control. On the side table of sofa there also lays a universal DVD recorder. Left screen shows your future, right one the past and the central screen shows your present.

Switch on the central screen, it shows your present sickness. Accept that many people suffered from this illness, you are not alone. Now switch on the right screen to see if you suffered from similar illness in the past. And if you suffered, then how did you treat it. Usually we don't find solution of current problems in the past. Now you minimize and freeze the past screen with remote control. Also, minimize and freeze the present screen.

Now relax and switch on future screen and try to find a solution to your problems. Now visualize a situation where you look perfectly healthy and your tumor has already dissolved. For example if you suffer from bone sarcoma in your thigh and can't even walk due to this illness; you may imagine that you are skiing in Switzerland. Feel the snow peaks, cold breezes, your friend's laughter, your own respiration sounds. Magnify these images, even increase brightness and contrast, and feel the reflection of these images on your body.

You may go to screen room daily, whenever you get time and see yourself skiing. Now you need not to view central and right screen any more. Directly start left screen, our next job is to record this skiing video on universal DVD recorder. The universal DVD recorder will relay this broadcast to the whole world. Your all nears and dears will know about your dream and start helping you to achieve this. To conclude the session, come out of the house and return to the river. Count up to seven and slowly open your eyes. Take a deep breath. This ends your visualization. Always keep in mind that the end should always be happy for everybody; nobody should be harmed any way.

Renovate your dream house if needed

You can construct some extra rooms in this house, if there is a need. For example you can make a small room for rest and relaxation. If you have some pain then you go to this room to relax for a while. You can also make a meeting room. You can invite here some important person to discuss your problem. For example you can call Dr. Johanna Budwig. You can sit with her, discuss and ask her opinion to solve your problem.

You can also invite your friends and close relatives to celebrate your successful skiing expedition. Imagine you are standing on the dice and narrating your experiences and everybody is clapping. The main essence of the story is that in the end people see you are healthy and cheerful. So that they also help you achieve your healthy and happy future. One question is very frequently asked is that how many times you should go to this house. Lothar says that there is no fixed rule but whenever you get time you should visit this house, may be twice a day. If the problem is serious then it is better you go there several times a day.

Visualization wonderfully brings positive changes in your health. It costs nothing but works 100%. You can use this treatment to heal your cancer, make your life happy and cheerful or even to just become a millionaire (Hirneise, 530).

Testimonials

Testimonials collected by **Cliff Beckwith**, a 15 year prostate cancer survivor "thanks to taking flax seed oil and cottage cheese", compiled & prefaced by healingcancernaturally.com.

Lung cancer healing testimony 1

Saturday Aug 19, 2000 I had a call from Casper, WY, that was exciting. The caller told me that in March, 2000 he was diagnosed with a serious cancer in his right lung and told that he did not have more than 1 to 3 months to live.

He was given chemo and couldn't stand it. He used morphine patches in case the pain got too great. He was 73 and had just about decided to go to the hospital and die.

At this point a rancher friend who had gotten a tape on Flaxseed Oil at a Bible conference heard about his situation and gave it to him. He told me he listened to the tape and fell in love with what he heard and immediately began to use 6 tablespoons of flaxseed oil and cottage cheese a day.

He said it "kicked in" right away, though usually it does not work quite that quickly.

He had an appointment with the Oncologist before long and the doctor took X-rays. The caller said he came out of the lab soon with a puzzled look on his face and asked him what, if anything, he had been doing.

He told the doctor he had been using flaxseed oil.

The doctor said that the tumor he had in his right lung had not changed, but the tumor in his left lung, about which he had not told him, had completely disappeared without a trace.

He gave the doctor a tape and told me that the doctor and nurses were making tapes and distributing them.

The caller said he was feeling good, continuing on the flaxseed oil and getting along well and seemed quite excited; as I was to hear it.

We are praising The Lord for His provision.

Lung cancer testimonial 2

A lady about 73 lived two houses down from us. She was a frail person and a smoker.

The doctors found a tumor about the size of a quarter on the lower part of her right lung and immediately urged an operation to remove half of the lung.

She was afraid she could not stand the operation and her grandson who knew us well urged her to go on Flax Oil. I talked to her as well.

She did but did not use it as she should have. Nevertheless there was no further growth of the tumor and I thought all was well.

About two years later I heard that she had died. Her grandson told me that on later checkups there was no growth of the cancer but the doctor kept urging an operation. The daughter that lived one door down did not want her to do it but she had five other children and they persuaded her to go along with the doctor's advice.

She did not make it off the operating table. The grandson did not feel kindly toward his aunts and uncles but rationalized that it was his Mamaw's time to go.

Lung cancer healing testimony 3

About 6 years ago a friend of ours had a cousin who was a veteran of World War II. He had very serious lung cancer and it had spread to his upper arm.

He got started with Flax Oil and it was not many months before we heard he was cancer free in a check up at the VA hospital. He called me and talked about it and was a happy man.

About two years later I heard that he had passed away. Some folks have the idea that flax oil is like an antibiotic. He got well so he saw no further use for the oil. That is a mistake. One should have at least a maintenance dose of oil each day to keep healthy.

He didn't and the cancer redeveloped. He decided that since it hadn't cured him he wouldn't bother with it again.

Lung cancer healing testimonial 4

The brother in law of Betsy, a member of a local church was 47 years old and incapacitated with lung cancer. This was around 7 years ago as I remember.

He had been given up and was doing no standard treatment. He began using 4 tablespoons of Flaxseed Oil a day with cottage cheese and in time [I do not know exactly how long but it was not many months] the only souvenir left was a little scar tissue and he was back at work. I never knew his name but did not about him. Betsy is the best friend of a good friend of ours.

I visited the church occasionally as the main musician was a fellow teacher and good friend. Kim was also the pastor's niece.

The pastor's wife had colon cancer and had part of the colon removed and had been put on heavy chemo. Kim wanted her to switch to flax oil but a daughter was a student nurse, and told her "Momma, do what the doctor tells you". In a while the lady had virtually no immune system left and the doctor advised her to stay away from people lest she catch a cold and die and took her off the chemo to see if her body could rebuild. Now she began using Flax Oil. In a short time the white count was going up and she was able to be out in public again. She had an appointment with the doctor and told him what she was doing. He told her that had not done her any good. It was the chemo that was helping her. She was put back on chemo and in about three months she went into a coma and died. The chemo had destroyed her heart and liver.

One Sunday night the pastor, John, asked me for a tape. I didn't know he had not had one. A few weeks later I visited again and was talking with John after the service. He told me that he hoped I was wrong but that he believed I was right. He said,

"They killed my wife". Then I asked him if he had heard about Betsy's brother in law. He said, "I hear he's pretty bad." I said, "He's well." Betsy was still there and John asked her how her brother in law was doing. She said, "He's well".

John looked at me, and with all the feeling he could put in it, he said, "There's going to be doctors in HELL because of things like this!!"

The average oncologist is doing the best he or she knows to do. The Hierarchy is another story as far as I can see. If flaxoil/cottage cheese were to be recognized officially as effective it would kill the profitability of the Oncology industry.

Cliff

Lung cancer testimony 5

Last June a friend of ours from beekeeping stopped by. She is a heavy woman, probably over 250 lbs. She had been diagnosed with a rapidly growing cancer in her lung.

The doctor was really after her to get it cut out as soon as possible. She was resisting because she did not think she could stand the operation. She began using 8 tablespoons of flax oil a day [which would be too much I believe if it were kept up] and in a checkup 8 weeks later there had been no further growth. The doctor still urged her to get an operation. A subsequent X-ray showed no growth but was a little fuzzy as to any reduction. She had an MRI Oct. 19 and a consultation Oct 25 but I haven't heard any results.

In January 2002 I learned that in early November of 2001 she had had a hip bone "explode" and had been hospitalized for quite a while, I think in late January before she was released. She did not have an opportunity to use the flaxoil/cottage cheese during that time.

She told me that the mass was still there but seemed to have changed its character. The doctor at that time did not believe it was malignant any longer but didn't want to go in and take anything for a biopsy as she was afraid she might bleed to death.

Today, June 30, 2002 I received word that she had passed away. I had not known any further details.

September 11, 2002 I received further word. The cancer had come back. She had gone back to the flaxoil/cottage cheese. At the time of her death the cancer had been eliminated except for two small spots in a lung and one in her liver.

She passed away as the result of ill health connected with Diabetes. A friend emphasized that it was not the cancer.

Lung cancer testimonial 6

About three years ago I was in my doctor's waiting room when a couple came in. I spoke to them briefly.

That night the lady called and told me that her husband was a retired college professor, 73, who had an 85% involvement with cancer in his left lung. The decision had been made to remove the lung at the Thompson Cancer center in Knoxville, Tn.

When the attempt was made it was determined that the cancer had spread further and they simply closed up and decided to use radiation and chemo.

The radiation had been done with no apparent results and he and his wife decided that rather than go through the misery of chemo they would just live as long as possible and forget it.

The oncologist did not argue with that. She suggested that they come to Rutledge and get flax oil and get started with four to eight tablespoons a day with cottage cheese.

They decided on 6 and got two quarts and then got their own after that.

Three months later I was in again and asked if she had seen him again. She had seen him the previous week. The cancer was still there but he was holding his own.

I remembered him about a year and a half later and she said that he had died, but that he did not die of cancer. He was not a very active person and died of a blood clot that moved to his heart.

Lung cancer testimony 7

I was diagnosed with stage IV lung cancer in January 2002. In March 2002 I had surgery and a nodule and the lower right lobe of my lung was removed. Five remaining nodules in both lungs. I began Iressa which is a oral cancer drug taken by mouth. At the same time I started taking 4 Tablespoons of flaxseed oil with one half cup of cottage cheese daily. When my cancer was diagnosed I was given three months to live. I am now close to my two year anniversary and while I cannot discount the Iressa I take daily, I give most of the credit to the flaxseed oil and cottage cheese. While on a trip to Oregon, I was unable to get lactaid free cottage cheese and did not take it for two weeks and experienced severe chest pains. They stopped when I resumed my daily regimen of oil and cheese. I am convinced it is what keeps me feeling wonderful and I do not even know I have lung cancer. Doctors who treat me and friends who observe me say they cannot believe that I have lung cancer either.

Beverly Christensen

Lung cancer testimonial 8

(sent to a Budwig support group on 23 August 2005)

I have endometrial adenocarcinoma stage IV now metastatic to lungs. My many tumors between the lungs have not grown since starting on the [nearly entire] Johanna Budwig protocol 8 months ago. I discontinued chemo last fall (my decision) as I knew I would not survive another treatment. Radiation and surgery are not options, per the doctors. Now my doctors say, "there is no medical explanation for why you are here".

I feel and look great!

If [someone] has been given a dismal diagnosis, he/she has nothing to lose by trying the Budwig Protocol.

Lung cancer testimonial 9

(sent to a Budwig support group on 4 October 2006)

A friend of mine was diagnosed on August 4, 2006 with lung cancer, stage 4 with mets to the rib and to lumbar #1. They also discovered a tumor measuring 2.8cm x 3.4cm on his lung. In addition, there were many tiny tumors forming around the large tumor. The oncologist started him on chemo.

By early September (7th which was a Thursday), I found out about my friend's condition and got the wife interested in the Budwig Protocol. As soon as she put the phone down, she rushed over to my house to get her first batch of flaxoil and cottage cheese and flaxseeds. I told her how to prepare it ...

She has been giving her husband 6 tbsp of flaxoil daily (plus the appropriate cottage cheese) since Sept 7. She has also changed the household food menu (no sugar, no cooked oils, no meat other than the occasional fish which is steamed or boiled, lots of fruits and fresh juices). A few weeks after taking on the Budwig Protocol, the husband began to regain some of his strength and was able to drive himself around again.

Last Monday (Oct 1), we spoke on the phone. They had just come back from a CT scan. The results were outstandingly good. The tumor size is down to 1.8cm x 3cm. There is also a clearing of the area around the tumor. As for the mets, it hasnt spread beyond those areas in August.

We are all stunned with the results ...

(http://www.healingcancernaturally.com)

Laetrile Testimonials

(From Dr. Binzel book "Alive And Well")

Case No. 14: T.P.

This 59-year-old man that was seen for the first time on 7/18/80. His history was that one month prior to this a routine x-ray showed a mass in his right lung. A biopsy showed this to be carcinoma. Five radiation treatments were given followed by one chemotherapy treatment that made him so ill he discontinued that whole program. He was started on my nutritional program.

An x-ray done in January, 1981, showed that the tumor in his right lung was completely gone. Let me quote from a letter I received from him on January 23, 1981:

"They were surprised here at [hospital name omitted] comparing the x-ray of last June and the one I just received .... Hope you understand what I am trying to say. I was really tickled when I learned the tumor was gone, and I thought of you right away. I know in my heart it was the Amygdalin and will never think differently.

"The doctor I had at the hospital in June said it was probably the 5 radiation treatments I had. They just don't want to admit [it was the Amygdalin], I guess."

My last contact with this patient was in April, 1993. At that time he was doing very well.

Case No. 21: E.D.

This 57-year-old man was first seen on 4/28/92 (and for that reason is not included in my statistical study) with a history of a diagnosis of carcinoma of the left lung 10 months previously. Surgery had been done followed by one chemotherapy treatment. This made him so ill that he discontinued it. He was then given 25 radiation treatments ending in December, 1991. In March,

1992, x-rays showed extensive growth of the tumors in that lung. He was placed on a nutritional program.

X-rays done in July, 1993, showed no further growth of the tumors in the left lung. X-rays done in November, 1993, showed that the tumors had all become scar tissue. In the most recent letter I received from him he stated that he was feeling so well that "I have no right to complain, so I have to cuss a lot about taxes, politicians, etc."

These statistics and case histories have focused primarily upon the extension of the patient's life span. That's certainly important, but the quality of life is also important. We will deal with that issue next.

The Budwig Diet quotes

"What she (Dr. Johanna Budwig) has demonstrated to my initial disbelief but lately, to my complete satisfaction in my practice is: CANCER IS EASILY CURABLE, the treatment is dietary/lifestyle, the response is immediate; the cancer cell is weak and vulnerable; the precise biochemical breakdown point was identified by her in 1951 and is specifically correctable, in vitro (test-tube) as well as in vivo (real)... "

Dr. Dan C. Roehm M.D. FACP (Oncologist and former cardiologist) in 1990

"Cancer patients suffer from a faulty metabolism caused by a malfunction in the lipid defense system. By repairing the lipid defense system the cancer cannot survive. Of course common chemo and radiation causes further harm to the lipid defense system -- the very system that protects you from cancer! The folks who will READILY ADMIT that they don't understand the cancer mechanism will tell you with their next breath that cancer can be killed with poisons. So can you. Would you trust your car to a so-called mechanic who didn't understand what makes a car work properly? If not, why would you let someone who doesn't understand cancer "fix" your body? The average cancer docs don't know - they admit it. That doesn't make them bad people; it just makes them unqualified to treat your condition if you have cancer. Don't let unqualified people poison you just because they don't know what else to do".

William Kelley Eidem, author "The Doctor Who Cures Cancer (Dr Revici)

"To sell chemotherapy as 'therapy' is most likely the biggest deceit in the history of medicine. Whoever masterminded this chemo-torture deserves a monument in the hell."

Dr. Ryke Geerd Hamer

"I have the answer to cancer, but American doctors won't listen. They come here and observe my methods and are impressed. Then they want to make a special deal so they can take it home and make a lot of money. I won't do it, so I'm blackballed in every country."

Dr Budwig

Dr Rudin believes the Omega 3 story parallels the story of Beriberi & Pellagra. It took them 200 years to accept pellagra was a nutrient deficiency.

"Nobody seemed to notice that a crime has been committed: It was the case of the missing nutrient. The nutrient was essential; it was a nutrient we human beings needed in order to stay healthy. It started to disappear from our diet about 75 years ago and now is almost gone. Only about 20% of the amount needed for human health and well-being remains. The nutrient is a fatty acid so important and so little understood that I call it "the nutritional missing link"....Food grade linseed oil & fish oil are the best sources of this special fat—Omega 3 essential fatty acid—which modern food destroys."

Donaldo Rudin, M.D. (The Omega 3 Phenomenon)

In a 1994 study of 121 women with breast cancer, those in more advanced stages whose breast cancer had spread to their lymph nodes showed the lowest levels of omega-3 fatty acids in the breast tissue. After 31 months, the 20 women who had developed metastases had significantly lower levels of these EFAs (Essential fatty acids) than those who didn't. Another study out of Boston University using the same type of tissue profiles that were used in the breast cancer study demonstrated that patients with coronary artery disease likewise had low levels of EFAs.

"The association between fats—meaning saturated, refined w6s (Omega 6), rancid fats, processed oils, and altered fats---and cancer, (but excluding w3s and fresh, natural, unrefined oils) has long been documented. (They) interfere with oxygen use in our cells. Heat, hydrogenation, light, and oxygen produce chemically altered fat products that are toxic to our cells....These fats kill people. Healing fats in cancer include...... Omega 3s, enhance oxygen use in cells, decrease tumor formation, slow tumor growth, decrease tumor formation, decrease the spread of cancer cells (metastasis), and extend the patient's survival time. Unsaturated fatty acids in fresh, unheated oils are anti-mutagenic. Saturated fatty acids to not have this protective ability. Heating these oils above 150^0 C makes them lose their protective power, and they become mutation-causing. ALL mass market oils except virgin olive oil have undergone heating during deodorization...When we use virgin olive oil or other unrefined oils for sautéing; frying...we overheat them, destroying their protective, anti-mutagenic properties. ALL hydrogenated and partially hydrogenated products have also been overheated.."

Udo Erasmus (Fats That Heal, Fats That Kill)

"Our immune system, which is vital for destroying cancer cells, requires EFAs, vitamins C, B6, and A, and zinc to function, and requires an exceptionally rich nutrient supply of ALL essential nutrients for its high level of complex cellular activities. Deficiencies of EFAs and toxic, man-made synthetic drugs that interfere with essential fatty acid functions can create the conditions of fatty degeneration collectively known as cancer."

Udo Erasmus

"Compared to 100 years ago, Omega 3 is down 80%, B vitamins are estimated to be down to about 50% of the daily requirement. Vitamin B6 consumption may be low as it is removed in grain milling and not replaced. Vitamins B1, B2, B3 and E have also been lost in food processing. Minerals are depleted in a similar way. Fiber is down 75-80%. Ant nutrients have increased substantially---saturated fat, 100%; cholesterol, 50%; refined sugar nearly 1000%; salt up to 500%; and funny fat isomers nearly 1,000%."

Dr Rudin

Dr. Johanna Budwig is rightly known far beyond the borders of Germany. Her ingenious, simple, and effective oil-protein diet has found adherents throughout the world and it has helped many people to particularly better deal with their cancer illness.

I had the great good fortune of spending many days in discussion with her over a period of several years, of being able to study her extensive case histories, of giving joint presentations with her, and of thus gaining an understanding of nutrition for myself that extended far beyond that which I was previously able to find in the usual literature. But what was most convincing to me in my activity on the executive board of Menschen gegen Krebs in Germany was the oil-protein diet.

Hardly a day goes by when I do not talk with people on the phone that has changed their diet along the guidelines provided by Dr. Budwig. I am party first-hand to how successful this nutrition therapy is. I consciously use the term nutrition therapy and not cancer diet because I think it would be an injustice to Dr. Budwig to not to distinguish her scientifically grounded oil-protein therapy from all the diets that are offered around the world.

For me the oil-protein diet always serves as the basis of a cancer therapy and please understands that I am not just simply writing this, but that I have carefully chosen my words, as I have become familiar with more than 100 different alternative cancer therapies in recent years, and I have investigated many of them. When Dr. Johanna Budwig died the cancer scene lost one of the last great scientists of the last century, and it behooves each of us to carry her legacy to future generations, so that they as well can profit from the oil-protein diet.

Lothar Hirneise

I am referring to a super nutrient, which has been neglected for decades, it is neither taught properly in the schools, nor the doctors discuss about it openly, multinationals have removed this from our diet, but the hard truth is that it is essential for our body, it keeps us healthy and fit, protects us from many serious ailments, its presence is essential for cellular respiration, our cells suffocate in its absence, without this our life is impossible, name of this nutrient is alpha-linolenic acid, which is head of the omega-3 family and the richest food source is FLAX SEED OIL.

Dr. O.P. Verma, Flax Guru

They (American Cancer Society) lie like scoundrels.
M. Dean Burk PhD who worked for the National Cancer Institute for 34 years

There have been many cancer cures, and all have been ruthlessly and systematically suppressed with a Gestapo-like thoroughness by the cancer establishment.

Robert C. Atkins MD

Essiac Is A Cure For Cancer. I've seen it reverse and eliminate cancers at such a progressed state that nothing medical science currently has could have accomplished similar results. I wouldn't have believed it myself had I not seen it with my own eyes. I feel very strongly that Essiac is the single most beneficial treatment for cancer today.

C.A. Brusch, M.D., J.F.K's personal physician talking to radio talk show host and producer Elaine Alexander in a radio broadcast from Vancouver, British Columbia, in November 1984

The War Against Quackery is a carefully orchestrated, heavily endowed campaign sponsored by extremists holding positions of power in the orthodox hierarchy.....The multimillion-dollar campaign against quackery was never meant to root out incompetent doctors; it was, and is, designed specifically to destroy alternative medicine...The millions were raised and spent because orthodox medicine sees alternative, drugless medicine as a real threat to its economic power. And right they are...the majority of the drug houses will not survive.

Dr Atkins, M.D. (The Healing of Cancer by Barry Lynes)

And what do I actually do? I give cancer patients simple, natural foods. That is all. I take sick people out of the hospital, when it is said there that they do not have more than an hour or two left to live, that the scientifically attested diagnosis is at hand and that the patient is completely moribund. In most cases I can help even these patients quickly and conclusively.

Dr. Johanna Budwig, in "Flax Oil as a True Aid"

Cancer has only one prime cause. It is the replacement of normal oxygen respiration of the body's cells by an anaerobic (i.e., oxygen-deficient) cell respiration.

Dr. Otto Warburg, twice Nobel Laureate

...the cause of cancer is no longer a mystery; we know it occurs whenever any cell is denied 60% of its oxygen requirements.

Cancer, above all other diseases, has countless secondary causes. But, even for cancer, there is only one prime cause. Summarized in a few words, the prime cause of cancer is the replacement of the respiration of oxygen in normal body cells by a fermentation of sugar. All normal body cells meet their energy needs by respiration of oxygen, whereas cancer cells meet their energy needs in great part by fermentation. All normal body cells are thus obligate aerobes, whereas all cancer cells are partial anaerobes.

Dr. Otto Warburg Prime Cause and Prevention of Cancer

[C]hemotherapy is basically ineffective in the vast majority of cases in which it is given.

Ralph Moss, PhD, former Director of Information for Sloan Kettering Cancer Research Center

Three Australian oncologists - Associate Professor Graeme Morgan, Professor Robyn Ward and Dr. Michael Barton - undertook a meta-analysis aiming to determine the actual contribution of cytotoxic chemotherapy to survival in adult cancer patients. Their results, published in "Clinical Oncology" in 2004 under the title "The contribution of cytotoxic chemotherapy to 5-year survival in adult malignancies" (abstract available at www.ncbi.nlm.nih.gov/pubmed/15630849) found the overall contribution of these drugs to 5-year survival in adults to be an estimated 2.3% in Australia and 2.1% in the USA. See Table: Impact of cytotoxic chemotherapy on 5-year survival in American adults showing the percentage of 5-year survivors after chemotherapy for 22 types of cancer. The authors concluded that "it is clear that cytotoxic chemotherapy only makes a minor contribution to cancer survival".

A detailed review of this important paper is owed to Dr. Ralph Moss and can be read for instance at www.icnr.com/articles/ischemotherapyeffective.html under the title "How Effective Is Chemo Therapy?"

Healing Cancer Naturally

"Best book I've ever read on chemotherapy."

Ralph Moss' Questioning Chemotherapy is a book that every person faced with cancer must read before submitting to toxic chemicals which may very well destroy the body's immune system. Unlike many alternative health authors who base their conclusions on anecdotal evidence, Moss uses the medical establishment's own research to prove that in almost all instances chemotherapy is NOT a viable approach to improving cancer survival rates. Moss also makes the important point that current cancer research has never bothered to examine the mental anguish, physical suffering, and poor quality of life endured by almost everyone whose doctors talk or scare them into undergoing chemotherapy. Learning about the economics behind chemotherapy drives the final nail into the coffin of a "therapy" that educated people in the future will consider outrageous and reflective of the current dark ages of so-called modern medicine. This is a must read book for anyone who wants to know the truth behind chemotherapy or anyone whose doctor wants to inject toxic chemicals into their bloodstream.

Chet Day's review of "Questioning Chemotherapy: A Critique of the Use of Toxic Drugs in the Treatment of Cancer" by Ralph W. Moss

Except for two forms of cancer, chemotherapy does not cure. It tortures and may shorten life...

Dr. Candace Pert, Georgetown University

Chemo drugs are some of the most toxic substances ever designed to go into a human body, their effects are very serious, and are often the direct cause of death. Like the case of Jackie Onassis, who underwent chemo for one of the rare diseases in which it generally has some beneficial results: non-Hodgkin's lymphoma. She went into the hospital on Friday and was dead by Tuesday.

Dr Tim O'Shea in TO THE CANCER PATIENT

Cancer researchers, medical journals, and the popular media all have contributed to a situation in which many people with common malignancies are being treated with drugs not known to be effective.

Dr. Martin Shapiro UCLA

~~**~~

Disclaimer

This book is not intended to replace the advice and/or care of a qualified health care professional. Please do not try to self diagnose or self treat any disease. Seek professional help and consult your physician before making any dietary changes.

This book is not intended to provide medical advice and is sold with the understanding that the publisher and the author have neither liability nor responsibility to any person or entity with respect to loss, damage or injury caused or alleged to be caused directly or indirectly by the information contained in this book or the use of any products mentioned. Readers should not use any of the product discussed in this book without the advice of a medical profession.

The Food and Drug Administration has not approved the use of any of the natural treatments discussed in this book. This book, and the information contained herein, has not been approved by the Food and the Drug Administration.

My Books

Cancer - Cause and Cure
Based on Quantum Physics developed by Dr. Johanna Budwig

http://www.amazon.com/Cancer-Quantum-Physics-developed-Johanna-ebook/dp/B00P3Y7BYG

Book Description

***** A must have book for every cancer patient *****

This book provides an introduction of Dr. Budwig's cancer research and treatment. Johanna Budwig (1908-2003) was nominated for the Nobel Prize seven times. She was one of Germany's leading scientists of the 20th Century, a biochemist and cancer specialist with a special interest in essential fats.

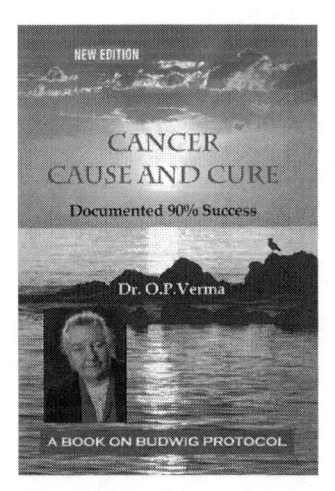

Otto Warburg proved that prime cause of cancer oxygen-deficiency in the cells. In absence of oxygen cells ferment glucose to produce energy, lactic acid is formed as a byproduct of fermentation. He postulated that sulfur containing protein and some unknown fat is required to attract oxygen in the cell.

In 1951 Dr. Budwig developed Paper Chromatography to identify fats. With this technique she proved that electron rich highly unsaturated Linoleic and Linolenic fatty acids were the undiscovered mysterious decisive fats in respiratory enzyme function that Otto Warburg had been unable to find. She studied the electromagnetic function of pi-electrons of the linolenic acid in the membranes of the microstructure of protoplasm, for all nerve function, secretions, mitosis, as well as cell break-down.

This immediately caused lot of excitement in the scientific community. New doors could open in Cancer research. Hydrogenated fats, including all Trans fatty acids were proved as respiratory poisons.

Then Budwig decided to have human trials and gave flaxseed oil and quark to cancer patients. After three months, the patients began to improve in health and strength, the yellow green substance in their blood began to disappear, tumors gradually receded and at the same time the nutrients began to rise. This way Dr. Budwig had found a cure for cancer. It was a great victory and first milestone in the battle against cancer. Her treatment protocol is based on the consumption of flax seed oil with low fat cottage cheese, raw organic diet, mild exercise, and the healing powers of the sun. She treated approx. 2500 cancer patients during a 50 year period with this protocol till her death with over 90% documented success.

She was nominated 7 times for Nobel Prize but with a condition that she will use chemotherapy and radiotherapy with her protocol. They did not want to collapse the 200 billion dollar business over night. She always refused to support the damaging chemo and radio for the sake of humanity.

Lothar Hirneise is founder and President of People Against Cancer, Germany. He travels a lot in search of finding most successful alternative cancer therapies. He has been student of Dr. Johanna Budwig. He is a great researcher and writer on alternative healing. He is successfully treating thousands of cancer patients at his 3-E center in Germany. In the last few years he has interviewed several hundred final stage so-called survivors, meaning patients who were in the final stage of cancer and who are all healthy again today. Based on his findings he proposed a 3 E Program – The Mnemonic of Cancer Treatment.

1) Eat well
2) Eliminate
3) Energy

He noticed that 100% of all survivors, did the energy work. In approximately - say 80% of all patients, had changed their diet. And in at least 60% of all patients, took intensive detoxification rituals. This is the basis of his, so much talked about 3E Program for healing cancer.

Lothar Hirneise strongly supports holistic and spiritual approach and includes Visualization, Tumor Contract, Meditation, mild Yoga, Emotional Freedom Technique, Dr. Ryke Geerd Hammer's New German Medicine (Connection of unresolved stress and cancer), Detoxification techniques (Soda Bicarb bath, Epsom bath, Sauna, Colon Hydrotherapy, Coffee Enema etc.) in his 3 E Program.

The book also, describes about rare and miraculous herbs used in the treatment of Cancer like Turmeric, Black seed, Ginger, Mistle Toe, Aloe vera, Echinecea, Lobelia, Essiac Tea, Pau d'arco Tea, Dandelion, Milk Thistle.

~~**~~

Awesome Flax: A Book by Flax Guru

http://www.amazon.com/Awesome-Flax-Book-Guru-ebook/dp/B00PUUIR0K

Flax seed- Miraculous Anti-ageing Divine Food

What is Flax seed and how can it benefit me? I was faced with this question when I started hearing about Flax seed not long ago. It became a 'buzz word' in society and seems to be making great role in increased health for many. I wanted to join that wagon of wellness and so I researched until I felt satisfied that it could help me, too. Here are my findings.

Flax seeds are the hard, tiny seeds of Linum usitatissimum, the Flax plant, which has been widely used for thousands of years as a source of food and clothing. Flax seeds have become very popular recently, because they are a richest source of the Omega 3 essential fatty acid; also known as Alpha Linolenic Acid (ALA) and lignans. People in the new millennium may see Flax seed as an important new FOOD SUPER STAR. In fact, there's nobody who won't benefit by adding Flax seed to his or her diet. Even Gandhi wrote: "Wherever Flax seed becomes a regular food item among the people, there will be better health."

Flax seed contains 30-40% oil (including 36-50% alpha linolenic acid, 23-24% linoleic acid- Omega-6 fatty acids and oleic acids), mucilage (6%), protein (25%), Vitamin B group, lecithin, selenium, calcium, folate, magnesium, zinc, iron, carotene, sulfur, potassium, phosphorous, manganese, silicon, copper, nickel, molybdenum, chromium, and cobalt, vitamins A and E and all essential amino acids.

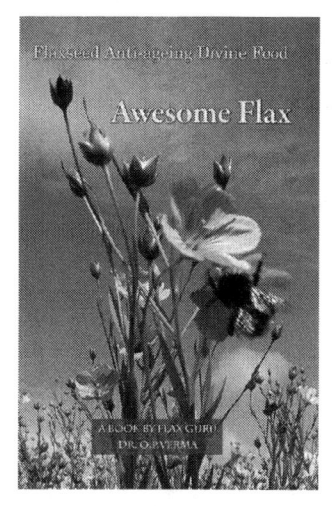

Other fatty acids, omega-6's, is abundant in vegetable oils such as corn, soybean, safflower, and sunflower oils as well as in the many processed foods made from these oils. Omega-6 fatty acids have stimulating, irritating and inflammatory effect while omega-3 fatty acids have calming and soothing effect on our body. Our bodies function best when our diets contain a well-balanced ratio of these fatty acids, meaning 1:1 to 4:1 of omega-6 and omega-3. But we typically eat 10 to 30 times more omega-6's than omega-3's, which is a prescription for trouble. This imbalance puts us at greater risk for a number of serious illnesses, including heart disease, cancer, stroke, and arthritis. As the most abundant plant source of omega-3 fatty acids, Flax seed helps restore balance and lets omega-3's do what they're best at: balancing the immune system, decreasing inflammation, and lowering some of the risk factors for heart disease.

One way that Omega 3 essential fatty acid known as Alpha Linolenic Acid ALA helps the heart is by decreasing the ability of platelets to clump together. Flax seed helps to lower high blood pressure, clears clogged coronaries, lowers high blood cholesterol, bad LDL cholesterol and triglyceride levels and raises good HDL cholesterol. It can relieve the symptoms of Diabetes Mellitus. It lowers blood sugar level. Flax seed help fight obesity. Adding Flax seed to foods creates a feeling of satiation. Furthermore, Flax seed stokes the metabolic processes in our cells. Much like a furnace, once stoked, the cells generate more heat and burn calories.

Flax seeds are the most abundant source of lignans. Lignans are plant-based compounds that can block estrogen activity in cells, reducing the risk of Breast, Uterus, Colon and Prostate cancers. According to the US Department of Agriculture, Flax seed contains 27 identifiable cancer preventative compounds. Lignans in Flax seeds are 200 to 800 times more than any other lignan source. Lignans are phytoestrogens, meaning that they are similar to but weaker than the estrogen that a woman's body produces naturally. Therefore, they may also help alleviate menopausal discomforts such as hot flashes and vaginal dryness. They are also antibacterial, antifungal, and antiviral.

Because they are high in dietary fiber, ground Flax seeds can help ease the passage of stools and thus relieve constipation, hemorrhoids and diverticular disease. Taken for inflammatory bowel disease, Flax seed can help to calm inflammation and repair any intestinal tract damage.

~~**~~

Secrets of Success: Smart way to success for every student

http://www.amazon.com/Secrets-Success-Smart-success-student-ebook/dp/B00Q3IIVAO/

Secrets of Success

Normally people think that memory, intelligence or learning ability is a God gift and it is not possible to further improve or increase the brain powers. We take it for granted that it will remain as it is gifted to us by God. But the truth is just opposite. Understand that as you go to gym for workout to develop your six pack abs, feed your body with muscle building food and get sharp sculpted body shape. Friends, believe me if muscle can be built and remodeled, then why not your brain's hardware and circuit boards. If you feed your brain with proper food it needs, follow simple instructions and take advantage of neurobics or mnemonics, you can immensely increase your brain's abilities.

We have tremendous powers locked inside our brains, but we are not using them to full extent. Dr. William James, considered the father of modern psychology, pointed out that "the average human being uses only 10 percent of his mental capacity." We still have to find out how much power or secrets are hidden in our brain.

Nowadays scientists have discovered mysterious techniques and nutrients to boost our brain powers. Today I shall raise curtains from all these secrets; I shall disclose all hidden tricks and tips. Today you are going to learn how your CPU, the brain tightly packed in a bony cabinet, functions. I teach you how each component and microprocessors works and how the best insulation material can be prepared. I also disclose the right technique to sharpen your brain and to make you an intelligent and successful scholar.

Today you will learn how to crack every examination you face, solve every question, defeat every opponent and get highest possible marks. You are going to write new equation of education and success.

Friends new boundaries and horizon of success is ready to welcome you. Today we shall discuss in detail about some great nutrients and supplements to boost your memory, learning, imagination, creativity and concentration. If you follow our suggestions and apply simple tricks you achieve a successful personality. This short e-book is going to prove a turning point in your life. Wish you luck.

Cancer Cure Is Found: Letrile is the answer

https://www.amazon.com/Cancer-Cure-Found-Laetrile-answer/dp/1797710206/

CANCER CURE IS FOUND

During 1950, a biochemist Dr. Ernest T. Krebs Jr., isolated a new vitamin from bitter apricot kernel that he called 'B-17' or 'Laetrile'. He conducted further lab animal and culture experiments to conclude that laetrile would be effective in the treatment of cancer. He proposed that cancer was caused by a deficiency of Vitamin B 17 (Laetrile, Amygdaline). Laetrile is a concentrated and purified form of vitamin B17. After a lot of research, he had finally developed a specific protocol to treat cancer. Laetrile Therapy combines Laetrile with nutritional supplements and a healthy diet to create a potent treatment that fights cancer cells while helping to strengthen the body's immune system.

Vitamin B-17, which is present in several different foods, consists of a locked substance which comprises two units' glucose, one unit benzaldehyde and one unit cyanide. When B17 comes in contact with a cancer cell it is unlocked by a hormone found only in the cancer cell, and becomes a lethal chemical bomb which destroys the cancer cell. Healthy cells do not cause breakdown of B17. Cancer is unknown to people living in areas with food products rich in B-17, and the population lives to a remarkably high age. Apparently nature has provided us with an ingenious defense against cancer, and it is an ordinary nutrient in our food. These are, amongst others nuts, seeds, vegetables, and in particular apricot kernels.

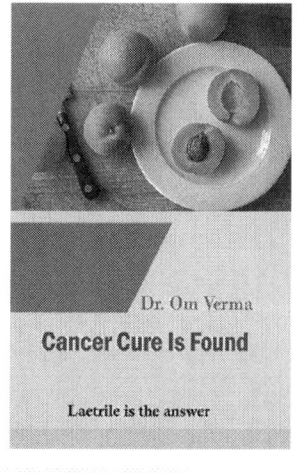

At present, patients listen or read a lot about Laetrile treatment, but usually they don't get precise and to the point information about what are the exact components of this protocol, where to get Laetrile injections and supplements, what to take, what not to take, what are the doses, how long to take the treatment, what diet they have to follow, etc. In this book, I have explained the protocol in detail proposed by Dr. Krebs. I have given every minute detail about Laetrile, other nutritional supplements and diet in this book. After reading this book patients can buy Laetrile injections, tablets and other nutritional supplements from the reliable sources (given in the book) and conduct the treatment under the supervision of their family doctor. Dr. Philip E. Binzel was personally trained by Dr. Ernest T. Kreb Jr. about everything of this treatment. Dr. Binzel had been using Laetrile therapy in the treatment of cancer patients since the mid 1970s. His record of success was astounding. Testimonies of his patients are also included in this book.

Made in the USA
Monee, IL
07 January 2020